No Retreat from Reason

AND OTHER ESSAYS

NO RETREAT
from
REASON

AND OTHER ESSAYS

———————

ALFRED E. COHN

KENNIKAT PRESS, INC./PORT WASHINGTON, N. Y.

To

RUTH

Contents

Preface

O F THESE essays, some are old and some new. The old ones have been much rewritten and modernized. What was said in general in the Preface of the old volume, called *Medicine, Science and Art: Studies in Interrelations* (University of Chicago Press, 1931) still expresses my sentiments. There is no need, therefore, for a new one.

Four essays on subjects related to the medical sciences which appeared in the collection of 1931 have been omitted from this book. "Purposes in Medical Research" (1924) served to introduce the *Journal of Clinical Investigation*. That publication was part of the medical contribution to the brave new world then in process of becoming. There have naturally been as many brave new worlds as there have been utopias to give expression to them. The successive stages in the development of medicine are part of the process. It reflects now the inescapable attempt to apply to this corner of human interest greater precision in observation and in classification and in the use of quantitative analytical methods in order to understand better the living processes which they illuminate. That effort is necessary in order to harness these processes to the rational will to understand.

A little later (1927) an address called "Medicine and Science" put forward the claim that even if diseases were accidents and no part of the *necessary* natural order, it is possible, nevertheless, to study these unfortunate phenomena, many of them avoidable, in precisely the same way that is employed in the effort to comprehend the inescapable manifestations of nature.

In the course of this general enterprise in medicine the claim of certain physiologists needed to be met that the processes of diseases differed from conventional physiological processes in nothing except differences of a quantitative nature. In "Physiology and Medicine" (1928) the problem, frequently met, was dealt with

which sought to make clear that a line exists at which a difference in quantity becomes a difference in quality. The point this essay emphasized is that this distinction needs to be made even when single variables alone are involved. Whoever has contemplated the subtle intricacies of a disease or, better, of a diseased person, knows that if the sum of his recognizable physiological parts is cast up the appearance he presents is still something qualitatively different from a mere quantitative heightening of a few specified living processes. He, or she, is a changed man or woman. Of course, in a disease, there is more or less of this or that. When a physiologist encounters it, he recognizes a novel situation and sends for a physician. In viewing nature, a change in the angle of vision of the spectator constitutes an element of importance. Clearly, many a discipline can try to absorb a near neighbor, but something, perhaps much, conceivably everything, can be lost in the process, the world being the poorer for the effort.

In the new medicine which the essay introductory to the *Journal of Clinical Investigation* described and defended, aspects developed which were not purely of a formal intellectual nature. Men were unavoidably part of this novel process. Soon there was strife. A man of medicine, in the era preceding, could, like Francis Bacon, preside over and know everything. That is what physicians had done. To be able to feel this claim, was a justifiable cause of pride. It is not so much that to master special forms of knowledge was necessary in the new medicine, though there are here also important deterring considerations, such as one's preferences and endowment, and that the day has a bare 24 hours. A man cannot do everything. To relinquish a possession or a vested interest without a struggle is a mutilating task. At least many a grand old man of medicine felt put upon. He resisted dislocation. And so there *was* strife. Being a man of peace I wrote "The Hierarchy of Medicine." I should now call that address (1929) delivered before the Alpha Omega Alpha Society in New York "Careers in Medicine." The object was to smooth ruffled feathers by pointing out that medical science and medical practice differed, as do physics and engineering, that to recognize this difference ought not to occasion grief, and that accepting this difference meant no loss in social stature. Time has been taking care of this controversy. So long as knowledge increases—and that means, temporarily, specialization—this situation, long unavoidable, will no doubt need always to be dealt with. Actors, not always steeped in historical wisdom, may be pardoned if it is not invariably possible for them to look out from between the upper and the nether millstones, the injuring pressure of which they cannot help feeling.

As for the essays, old and new, they are the off-thinkings of living the life of a medical scientist who has taken his living with seriousness not undiluted, he hopes, with humor. He is not less nor more content with the world than he was when he and it were younger. Freud and Marx had already galvanized us into apprehensiveness. That is all the more reason for setting down the reasons for mere dissatisfaction. Otherwise there would be nothing ahead but despair. Actually, there seems little reason for that; the trouble for most people now is not that there is new ugliness, though there is plenty of that, but that there is so much of it everywhere, the reports of the spread of this being brought daily to our door-step. But with the ugliness there is so much more new rational thinking devoted to curing the sick old world that the historically minded are, I think, justified in entertaining hope. It matters though. History is not just history. History it has been insisted upon more than once depends, in its recital, on a man's beliefs. He can be an evolutionist, a simple creature who watches what has evolved and tries to discover meaning—or a moralist who thinks he can discern purpose, perhaps because he thinks he knows what it is. For him it would be a great disappointment to learn it may not be about anything.

ALFRED E. COHN

The Hospital
The Rockefeller Institute for
  Medical Research

No Retreat from Reason

AND OTHER ESSAYS

Psychoanalysis in Medicine

WHETHER psychoanalysis belongs in the scheme of medical things has been a source of troubled searching on the part of the profession of medicine these many years past. Pride and prejudice have had their share in keeping the surface of the pure waters of science and research in a bemused but also a beruffled state. Psychoanalysis has been joyously acclaimed as the reconciler of many and diverse imaginings by men groping seriously for help in a corner of human experience, sadly and painfully disturbed, sadly in need of understanding themselves; and by others, read categorically out of the profession with very slight, short shrift. There are now in fact few men into whose ken has not come at least one man or one woman actually reborn or reconstituted by the new bewildering insight, few men who have not had occasion for thankfulness for the gift of this painful, but at the same time beneficent source of healing.

Perhaps it is an error to try to find a lineage for this child of 19th Century thought. Perhaps it did grow in a single generation in the consciousness of one or two master minds. Perhaps it is an error to search further afield for cognate relatives or to dig too conscientiously for forebears in a dimmer, distant past. But the sense of the concatenation of things, which perforce is strong upon us, breeds belief that somehow things have ancient causes and prods us on to an exploration of the Western mind with the hope that a legitimate parentage is to be found—that this offspring of its suffering has had an abiding respectability. If a rigorous systematizing genealogist were in the end to be unconvinced that the line of descent is pure rather than spurious, the adventure has had nevertheless a charm, not too much mitigated by the dangers of the chase.

Somehow, the place which we now seek, with a show of contentment, to assign to psychoanalysis has long had a precarious

3

footing. It is putting perhaps too fine a point on etymology to find in the word πσύχη the open sesame that links this current of our interest to ancient gropings intellectually of the most gracious, the most humane of our spiritual ancestors. But they had, when the imagination was fresh, bold, and adventurous, a keen awareness that somehow men possessed a supersensuous element of which we are so imminently aware as to feel the compulsion to treat it as if it were as real to our perceptions as are our sensuous experiences.

To lean in this fashion too heavily on the slender reed of etymology is, again perhaps, to follow too trustingly the call of that enticing will-o-the-wisp. The soul, or the conceptions of it, achieved an audacious, a checkered career, across the painful, romantic centuries of the Christian dispensation. After those years when the need for its cultivation was founded in the sensitive experience of a sensitive race, a new era, that of our own time, with a new and a different temper developed a requirement all its own for its recreation. It made of the soul something to be recognized no doubt but, as soon as recognized, to be relegated to the land of limbo, not knowing what place to assign to it in the material of a mechanistic world. Descartes had no wish to deny the soul, but for the purposes of his rational world he found no other disposition for it than, after the manner of the new rationalism, to pin a label on it and then not knowing what to do with so troublesome a member, to tuck it away inside the deepest recess of the cranium in the least conspicuous, the most hidden center of the brain. And there it lay, more than three centuries, until the very foundations of that world which decided not to trouble about its value began to crumble. In its troubled travail the search for the soul began again—more painfully, more tentatively, more realistically, more despairingly—because of the pain, the tenuousness, the reality, the despair of this world of ours, that began, as never before, because of its loneliness, to find a need to take counsel of the very deepest, the most inward awareness of our being.

How curious the behavior of Nemesis. She managed to bring home to us, very soon, the consequences of our historical misdeeds. Having substituted for an interest in the salvation of our souls, faith in the beneficence of material gain, she has taken advantage, speedily, of our lack of a sense of proper values and has visited upon us, almost as if it were punishment, a sickness of the soul— the very existence of which we were beginning to feel strong enough to deny.

Our pain is evident enough. To know that this suffering is self-inflicted does not lessen its severity. Nor is the sickness evenly distributed. Clearly the possessors of material things are being worse put to it than the poor and humble. Striving, we can now see, is more exhilarating than merely defending. Common men, caring for a better even if it is only a simple world, are evidently more robust of spirit than those for whom living has only the worth of possessing goods or of exercising power. The rescue of political, of social, of spiritual values, crushed by the weight of *things,* is becoming the crucial issue in the will to survive. These are the values which a hundred years of revolutionary experience have revealed as being the proudest of our possessions—the possession of our very selves—the value of those selves as units of a humane, a democratic, a generous society.

There was a world, the world of the Middle Ages, which this one of ours decided not wholly to inherit. Its span spread from the era of the *Sermon on the Mount* to a scarcely recognized death in that of the *Summa Theologica.* The thought dawned that the power of the mind should be asserted as superior to a power of the spirit. That mood became stronger. In the 17th Century it was so strong that Descartes could go so far as to dispense, in a scheme of things, even with the secondary characters of things, perceived by the senses, and came to rely for knowledge on primary qualities susceptible of proof by measurement. It was a glorious epoch, this new one, in which were accumulated that dominance over nature and those coins in coffers the very possession of which has created those partial dissatisfactions the expressions of which can now no longer be suppressed. Our nostalgia has not the sentimental cast of the 18th Century. The steel and iron of the machine have entered so the structure of our being that we think still to cure our ills by mechanisms. Mechanisms! How came it, that in this insistence on mechanism it was conceivable impotently to leave out of a mech-anistic universe what Descartes had so joyfully discarded. If the mind and the spirit were inescapable possessions what were their place in nature? Legitimately and illegitimately, thought, reason and experiment; charlatanry, pseudo-science; science and philosophy have all sought possible answers. Masters of religion, physicists like Sir Oliver Lodge, societies for psychical research, public men, great biologists, philosophers, General Smuts, Jacques Loeb, Professor Whitehead have all broken lances in the struggle to attain insight and exact understanding, each wielding his, powerfully, according to his lights, his comprehensions, his needs, his intentions. It has been a gallant struggle this—to seek to put the mind, the spirit, the soul, back into the body. Harvey Cushing, in the neat manner of a surgeon, put it back as a kind of principle of organic leadership into the pituitary gland, not far away from the pineal, where Descartes left it.

It remained for Sigmund Freud, adopting the technique of a scientist, to define and to isolate an aspect of this problem and to explore according to the methodology familiar to scientific enterprises, a set of phenomena, accessible to observation, subject to accumulation and classification and analysis. Motives, as these lay on the surface of consciousness, or deeply concealed in our all but inaccessible interior, became the objects of his explorations. He sought to discover the paths and by-paths which motives traveled in their careers of forming and influencing the content of our mind and our memory and of putting compulsions on the behavior of our kind. He chose a set of motives, arbitrarily perhaps, perhaps with erring insight, but perhaps faultlessly. It does not matter. What he proposed came pat to our need. What he devised was a way of exploration. Already a generation speaks his language and unconsciously thinks in patterns formed of his suggestion. The mind, or an important part of its activity, has become amenable to study.

That the mind has been rediscovered as an identifiable instrument which in its operations seems to obey a customary and orderly procedure, is an outstanding contribution of our time. It is striking that it began again to be explored just when the need for it, because it was sick, was becoming insistently patent. To wiser and more experienced hands must be left the business of describing mental or psychic mechanisms. What I can do is to bear witness and to testify that whatever its nature it operates in the body of which it is an integral part. It is no part of the purpose of this essay to take position on whether the two, mind and body, are two or one, separable or inseparable, cast in each other's image or working at cross purposes. And if working at cross purposes, this form of illness is different from that comparable mechanism, inside consciousness, when sickness comes on because the mind itself falls victim to conflict of motives within its own self.

The point of striking significance now concerns the rediscovery of the importance of the mind in the effort at understanding diseases, or certain of them, and has issued from the need to find whether there is a place in their progress for the operation of the mind because exploration on the basis of purely physical mechanisms was leading to no satisfactory solutions. Since the search for certain explanations along avenues simply mechanistic has become exhausted, the thought, or the need, to look elsewhere has suggested itself. To seek clues for certain ills in ways that the mind could reveal is not a new impulse. What is new is that that search has persisted into an epoch in which many men of great insight and knowledge, with the temper of scientists and trained in the methods of science, were concluding that mechanical operations no longer sufficed in the attempt at understanding all things. The good fortune of our time has consisted in pointing out how, methodologically, the search in new directions is to be conducted. Success is the better assured because of the need of the mechanistic enterprise itself, to seek psychological aid. It is as if a once strong brother found the aid of a weaker, a necessity. And mechanism is paying its debt for this aid by lending to psychological exploration its own indispensable methods of intellectual precision.

Now it cannot be the function of these remarks to be systematic. They cannot and they do not wish to be a catalogue. The phrase "psychological component" has become current to so great an extent as to be a cliché. It covers the situation in which, during a long or a short, clearly mechanistic illness, some sort of mental disturbance has supervened. The mental aberrations of cardiac and nephritic patients and of patients suffering from arterial hypertension are cases in point. It is used when a mental disturbance is intrinsic to the total appearance as in cerebral arterial affections of the aged, when physical and mental derangements come on simultaneously. It is often not sufficiently in evidence when emotional disturbance, of long standing or short, is the dominant ailment. In this category fall individuals who through shock or continued strain develop glycosuria, perhaps diabetes mellitus, or polyuria, or paroxysms of tachycardia, or recurring premature cardiac contractions. Cases of asthma, in which attacks are clearly associated with profound emotional disturbance, seem to belong in this group. How far mental or emotional disturbances can account for the development of diseases—even of infectious ones like tuberculosis—is not a problem which can be faced here. There are physicians, intelligent and sincere, who entertain this view of the origin of diseases like pneumonia or pulmonary tuberculosis. It is not one which, just now, commends itself; it goes further, it seems, than the obvious bits of knowledge we possess, permit. In situations in which long continued or brief mental disturbances develop, consequences often follow in disturbances of the performance of ordinary bodily functions. It is then that malfunction in gastric, urinary, circulatory, muscular and intestinal systems becomes manifest. These have very great importance because, weak creatures that we are, they offer us, even if they do not afford an opportunity for understanding, the chance, nevertheless, to embark on a therapeutic exploration. It is here beyond all other situations where bodily relief can be attained through understanding that mental processes have gone awry. Here the search for motive, for psychic injury, for social disharmony finds a most satisfactory reward.

But there has accumulated in the literature of this subject a mass of information in the form of well-observed cases which throw light on the situations and conditions in which, through exploring the behavior of the mind, an insight has been gained on the intricate interrelations of the mind and the body. What is striking is how many tissues, organs and systems are called upon, and in how many ways, to be surrogate for mental and emotional distress. Headaches, dyspnoea, palpitation, vomiting, glycosuria, polyuria, cyanosis, all constitute ways of expressing dissatisfaction. Not the least of the interesting inquiries which have been set in motion, concerns the possibility of dividing into classes, individuals who respond with dysfunction or hyperfunction or hypofunction of the particular structure which they employ, in fact, for the purpose of their protection.

But this is scarcely the place in which illustrative cases should be cited. They are to be found in many books and in articles in journals. They exhibit a wide range of convincingness. And that itself is evidence of the current state of knowledge. It is not a novel experience in empirical undertakings to find that an effort is made to attempt to fit a new proposal to an extensive gamut of occurrences—often so inclusive as to suggest a certain recklessness in the enterprise. No harm is done provided a sense of humor abides with us. Besides, at the beginning, whether a pattern fits a circumstance cannot always be known. In the interpretation of dreams and in many another bit of contributory evidence, that the plain meaning could be what it undoubtedly is seemed incredible or so very obscure and so remote from sensible understanding as to make it surprising but finally convincing that it made sense.

There has been no lack of warning as to what caution should be observed in so young a discipline, especially full of pitfalls on the part of wilful men. To utter warnings is necessary but also almost always futile. Men, in the presence of the unknown, do what they must. When the need is as great as it is in the domain of sane and gracious living, it is not difficult to excuse exuberance. It is in our own rescue that we tend to become reckless. For serious men this has been a brave adventure. The exposure of charlatans can be left to the good sense of the community—and to time. Not to try when trying is so full of promise, is to be timid when timidity, it is now clear for many a man and woman, spells disaster.

There can be doubt no longer that analysis of the operations of the mind, of behavior in general, has a necessary and so a legitimate place in the scheme of things. The search to find that place has occupied men in many walks of life—from medicine to politics. Finally, this way is full of high promise. It works, we think, because the pattern fits so often. And there is confidence in the manner of this working because in our time our confidence in the method has been so amply confirmed. If science, and the method of science, is not a way of life it is at least a way of looking at nature. And its way of looking at this corner begins to make sense—men and their fortunes begin to fall into categories. And these, as is so often the case in the scientific enterprise, take on configurations which recurrently are recognizable. Rules, even if not laws, emerge. Today we do not, but tomorrow we shall have deeper insights into the actual operation of this most important matter in life—the way of our thinking and feeling.

First published in 1941, the Institute for Psychoanalysis.

No Retreat from Reason

I F FREE men are to survive in a free society a retreat from reason is unthinkable. Only if free societies cease to exist, can the use of reason be abandoned. The choice, freedom or no freedom, is fundamental and anterior, and depends on what kind of life, in what kind of society, we choose to create. The choice cannot be made decently without experience—our own or that of others. In that background we exercise our choice. Nor can a choice be made successfully without the use of those powers given to us by nature. If we do not possess these powers the retreat from reason is not a choice but a necessity. One hundred and fifty years of history must have assured us that we can manage—that in some measure our abilities are equal to the demands on them—not without difficulty, not without danger. But danger is inescapable; it is the price of free choice, the price of reason.

I propose to argue that to reason it is essential to know what we are to reason about, that the only thing about which we can reason is this world, that after reason comes action—to go along with reason; or to retreat. I propose to examine the meaning of four words—reason, science, civilization, society. We are experienced enough to know that no word has the same meaning for all men. We must examine the meaning, therefore, of these words. I have chosen them because they symbolize, it seems, the storm centers about which the very proposal to retreat from reason rotates. Only free men, after they have faced the realities implicit in these meanings, can choose how to act. The misuse of that opportunity, you must be acutely aware, may turn into disaster.

Reason itself is, it is unnecessary to insist, merely a function of the mind. The use which is made of this instrument gives us no assurance that the result will constitute correct judgment or indeed only correct judgment. Reason is solely a technique for examining situations and ideas, of attempting to estimate aspects concerning them such as their inner consistency and their cogency. Reason itself does not choose the premises from which an argument flows. It attempts to see though that the flow makes sense. The premises of any society are the assumptions, the axioms, the postulates which underlie all our arrangements—derived in the first instance from the recollection of experience.

Because I am a medical scientist you will expect, correctly, that I shall be arguing for the positive value of science or at least for the value of its outlook and its method. But life is a whole. It is the sum of all the currents of our interests; these run through it, sometimes parallel, sometimes at angles. We do not lead scientific lives, and then social lives, and then economic lives and then political lives. We lead life as a whole, all these lives at the same time; if not, we lead it in such a way that life becomes confused and unbalanced. We cannot permit a minor current to deflect the whole stream. Science must fit into life.

If you read what is being written in increasing volume about how science is not doing enough to make available for everyone the social goods which it contributes, and read also about how many of its discoveries and advances turn out to be destructive to the very existence of human society, you must appreciate what is meant by making science fit into the whole pattern or scheme of life. The dangers into which science has been running society have caused thoughtful people, including scientists, to take alarm. How great a place science has come to occupy in communal life cannot escape anyone's observation. For example a knowledge of the intricate constitution of protein molecules will alter, sooner or later, more profoundly even than rayon has done, the entire silk industry and the lives of the great variety of persons on two continents at least, dependent upon it—from growers of silk worm cocoons to manufacturers and distributors of silk fabrics. Is this result the consequence of the application of a single simple scientific principle or scientific discovery? By no means. The final stage was taken by Carruthers in utilizing certain chemical properties of certain protein molecules. But the idea that that could be done rested on other investigations—painstaking and very time-consuming earlier discoveries of the arrangements and qualities of the constituent molecules with techniques like X-rays and the analysis of the structure of crystals. In the production of a pair of silk stockings, themselves wanted for intricate emotional and esthetic reasons, lie interconnected the lives of men, women and children, devoted to purposes apparently, but only apparently, as unconnected as seem to be the lives of physicists, chemists, agriculturists, manufacturers, financiers, builders, stevedores, sailors, real estate operators, and locomotive engineers. Where the work of a scientist, no matter how pure, ends, from the point of view of a society in which he flourishes, is a problem by no means simple to define. If the end result of the process, possessing a pair of silk stockings, were decided to be too unsubstantial a good to warrant waging a war, where, in the course of the very long train of events from chemist to manufacturer, is it possible to call a halt? Stop it at the level of research in protein chemistry, a level where you deal with relatively a simple organization of things, and you interfere with advances in knowledge issuing in improvements in genetics, in the manufacture of countless articles which have a use in peaceful pursuits—the making of foods, of clothing, of glassware, of drugs.

Obviously, scientists do not live unto themselves alone. Being parts of society, every act of theirs is reflected somehow in the course of the lives of other men. Desirable as it may be to put brakes on any of the processes of the living social organism, associations for the advancement of science seem likely to encounter difficulties almost insurmountable in separating what they decide to regard as socially desirable from things socially hostile. Difficult as the separation undoubtedly is, no one can look upon the chance of failure with equanimity. I mean to return to a further consideration of this problem. Science and scientists are embedded inextricably and very naturally and desirably in the matrix of the whole of our society. I am taking the view that the ties which bind science to life are inescapable and the influences which life exerts on scientists, determining.

Two views have been taken of the interrelation of science and society. The older view was held without challenge almost to our own day. It was the common impression that novelty in thought, invention in technology, discovery in science, depended on the initiative and thinking of private scholars. Unlike artists they had no private patrons—they performed what they were driven to perform in institutions of learning or, presumably, with resources of their own. Sight should not be lost though, of the opportunities and facilities placed at their disposal by the Academies and Learned Societies. These were fostered by rulers and the rich and powerful beginning in Florence with the Accademia del Cimento (1657-1667) as is so admirably narrated by Martha Ornstein (in *The Role of Scientific Societies in the Seventeenth Century*). To a large extent they may be regarded as having been private scholars. With few exceptions that day is all but gone. What they did, so ran the general belief, contributed somehow to the development of the social structure. The result was an aid to what was designated as progress. Because what they did seemed to make sense, in that one step led to another, logic, whatever that is, was supposed as a thread to run through their acts. It was also believed, no doubt more or less unconsciously, that what was contributed was motivated toward realizing what Aristotle would have called a final cause—an objective toward which, in the words of *In Memoriam,* "the whole creation moves."

In the absence of any other formulation, no one troubled particularly to explain how so random an attempt, or better no attempt, at orderliness was to achieve an unpremeditated desired end. The system seemed to work though there was no pattern to show how it did so—it required no one's thoughtful attention, it was a part, unrecognized and not understood, of the system of *laissez faire.*

It is well known that under many circumstances, in many environments, there are spirits who regard themselves as wholly free to think what they please, to pursue what interests them, to believe that a new direction of thought is, or can be, of their own making. This view is part of the conventional idea of the habit of genius. Genius works, not by passing stepwise slowly and painfully from point to point but by great leaps from lofty crag to lofty crag—without signposts, without evidence, without intervening stages but under the influence of what is called, roughly, intuition, itself a function, if it exists at all, vaguely understood. In point of fact in the evolution of ideas steps are taken but they are rather of a different nature, small though radical, such as Einstein described as involving the differences between Aristotle and Galilei regarding the nature of motion. Genius in short, at least in the more or less popular view, is a possession that permits sudden overturns in conception, or revealing expressions, in extraordinary form possessing extraordinary content. Newton and Shakespeare are our outstanding examples.

I think there can be no doubt—at least there is no reason for entering a discussion—that men can be wholly unconscious of any motive driving them to their acts outside their own volition. That, as I have said, is the traditional view. As a view, it has scarcely been contested until our own time. But recently, at the Second International Congress on the History of Science and Technology in London, in 1931, another view was offered by a Russian scholar interested in the history of science and the history of scientific ideas. His is an arresting notion. Serious students have not dismissed it. So weighty a scientific journal as *Nature* has devoted space to its analysis. Volumes on science, both natural and political, have since been published which profess to have been influenced by Professor Hessen's contention. More recently, in 1937, G. N. Clark, an Oxford scholar, reviewed Hessen's argument. He found in it, I think, no essential fault. He discovered errors in detail which cannot be regarded as seriously damaging. He has taken too narrow a view, however, of what is meant by the interaction of social influences and science. He has divorced more sharply than seems possible, personal motive from social motive, and economic motive from the totality of social interest and necessity. Hessen was analyzing the background and development of the thought of Isaac Newton. The correctness of all the details of the analysis need not concern us but for the purpose of this argument his general insight concerning the dependence of originality, even of men of genius, on the influence of the past and knowledge of the present is illuminating. The view is that Newton's interest in such problems as the general law of attraction, the tides, determining longitude, a lunar theory in gravitation, were no accident, but had their origin in compelling contemporary requirements, such as finding one's position at sea and in such other subjects as warfare and especially ballistics. Ballistics was important in the study of the trajectory of cannon balls. And cannon balls were important as a means of helping on the political and economic interests of the rapidly growing British empire. The degree of certainty with which it is possible to derive Newton's interest in this fashion is relatively unimportant, but of this one can be certain. However unformed the motives may have been and however inchoate the accumulations of natural knowledge, search for such knowledge was regarded as urgent. For this, founding the Royal Society, devoted to fostering advance in natural knowledge is good evidence. There was little doubt in the minds of the Fellows or in that of the British Government which gave the Society its charter in 1662, that its deliberations whether of pure or applied science were destined to give the commerce of Great Britain an advantage in the struggle for power in which the nation was already engaged. I can quote an observation of Bishop Sprat, the earliest historian of the Royal Society, to this end:

By their *naturalizing* Men of all Countries, they have laid the Beginnings of many great Advantages for the future. For by this Means, they will be able to settle a *constant Intelligence*, throughout all civil Nations, and make the *Royal Society* the general *Bank* and Free-port of the World: A Policy, which whether it would hold good in the *Trade* of *England*, I know not; but sure it will in the *Philosophy*.

Of this Society, Newton was a member.

In our own day there is further evidence for the view that scientific enterprise is not always a spontaneous movement but often has its origin in the deliberations of thoughtful and far-seeing laymen in efforts to plan for the welfare—and the warfare—of their communities. The many activities of the National Research Council in its several sections—on public health, the physical sciences and the social sciences are evidence how organization is provided on a national scale to substitute for haphazard reliance on genius. The extent to which the great philanthropic foundations propose, foster and support programs of research illustrates the same principle. The almost countless prizes for essays, scholarships and fellowships, research institutes, scientific expeditions, devoted to the advancement of knowledge in directions regarded as wise and desirable by donors and founders are eloquent evidence that the mind, unlike the wind, bloweth not always where it listeth. On the contrary it takes advantage often of the direction given to it by shrewd and far-calculating men.

In two senses, therefore, the very existence of the scientific enterprise suggests that the time is not ripe for retreat. Scientists push forward in purposeful directions and society, if scientists themselves were not ready to do so, would put pressure on them to see to it that they proceed with furthering the choice to which that society is committed.

Now the methods of science can easily be misunderstood. I have already explained how the subjects which are investigated originate, how they do not arise simply or solely in the imaginations of scientists. Scientists know more or less the histories of their subjects and receive suggestions there for further researches. Very frequently, especially in these latter days, the requirements of industry or the demands of national defense suggest to them what had best be done. What has surprised historians is how rarely forward steps are taken without traversing intermediate ground. There are, as I have said, no great leaps; there are no great primary originations. Implicit in a current situation is almost always something that has pointed the way, usually only a short way. It is one of the great hazards of the game that rarely, on looking forward, can there be any certainty that the step about to be taken is necessarily correct. The forward movement in science is usually tentative and is dependent on what is known as the technique of trial and error. In philosophy this is known as empiricism. Knowledge and a sense for possibility, narrowed to probability, are the aspects through which mental processes pass in attaining advanced positions. Knowledge and the need for reducing possible courses to probable ones involve the operation of reason—searching, testing, and discarding many methods and finally adopting a likely one. Unless the function of reason were orderly and were capable in some way of running parallel with and, in a sense, of testing its performances against the operations of nature, we might still be in the stage of witchcraft, alchemy, and astrology. In science, what we do in order to succeed must fit somehow into the processes of nature. Reason, the ability to select likely ways of accomplishment, goes a long way toward making possible solutions of value. Looking backward after a successful campaign, the elements which have facilitated the result have the air, even if they are known to have been selected haphazardly, of having fallen inevitably into place, so pat is the design. Unfortunately much of the history of discovery is written as if chance had played a minor role. Actually any candid investigator, who has the ability accurately to recapitulate the course of his thinking—and such men are rare—would confess to how checkered and how fortunate, how lucky, his course had been. To what extent reason takes part in this process is far from certain. It operates on proof. Experience is necessary. But experience may not be able to suggest what plan, in reason, must necessarily be followed. For this, the ways of nature are far too subtle. What can be asserted is that whatever is done, will subsequently conform to reasonable process.

I want to return to the phrase I regard as central to this discussion: reason is the operation which issues in choice—choice being witness that we have the opportunity and the obligation to behave as men who have and must shoulder responsibility. In this light I want next to examine the meaning of the word "civilization." In these days we are being told that this is something we are on the verge of losing—as if it were a substance, some concrete thing which exists in its own right, in a recognizable form, of which we are presumably actually possessed. But whether we have it or not, it is necessary to discover and to describe what the order is of the thing we hold so precious. The word is used to connote many situations—ancient and modern, Oriental and Western, European and American, Baltic and Mediterranean, Greek, Roman and medieval, Christian, Hebrew and Pagan. These words all denote civilizations. When we speak of losing our own, is it any of these we are losing, one or all or none, but instead something peculiar to ourselves, the product of our own manufacture? Is a civilization something which follows an already existing pattern, or a series of patterns, or is it an agglomeration, an accumulation, a deposit, fortuitous, unpremeditated, amorphous, like a paleolithic kitchen midden? Or is it just born, born spontaneously, or something that grows, or something that like one's clothes is made to suit—either a time, or a nation, or a people, or a climate? How do we recognize whether somewhere, at some time, there is or has been such a contrivance? Toynbee has been in process of writing nine volumes in which are to be accumulated specimens to which this word can be applied. Toynbee's is a very ingenious notion. If you can accumulate enough specimens you can examine them at leisure to study their construction and to see whether they contain elements common to them all. If you find a common thread you have a guide to their nature. You can then learn, perhaps, whether there is a course all of them follow, discover the respects in which they resemble one another and distinguish wherein they differ. To assemble the specimens means, of course, that a way exists of identifying them. That means, no doubt, possessing rough preliminary specifications to which all of them conform. To find the specimens is itself an exciting adventure as anyone who has entered upon it knows to his delight. To know that there are many has this importance— it assures us that we too can have one suited to our needs—that there is no ironclad inevitability about our own. Toynbee is not the only modern historian who has entertained himself with this fascinating search. Spengler's study suggests a related conception.[1]

[1] I have come to think of Toynbee's *A Study of History* from a different angle. The question has become: To what extent has Toynbee adhered to the method of science? It was necessary for him to define the "nature" of a society. His definition had perforce to be a deduction. In scientific method, induction follows deduction endlessly, each stage following inescapably a preceding one because of the discovery of new or further fact. In the study of history, that is not practicable; the record is scarcely sufficiently indisputable, despite Mommsen. Opinion enters the making of a definition. Correspondence to the definition chosen imposes a degree of arbitrariness on the shape, or the description, of the societies selected. The temptation to make an accommodating definition is naturally difficult to resist. Will, rather than patent fact, becomes, then, determining. That is not science.

Whether there is an historical process and what is the nature
of its mechanism has often enough been the subject of vigorous
and penetrating discussion. Its mechanism is far from having
always been regarded as identical. For some thinkers a civilization
is something like a play in five acts, having a beginning and a
middle and an end. With the last act the play ends. There is no
provision for a next play. There may not even be a next play. For
others, it has no end but passes to and fro from the rule of the
many to the rule of the few. Sometimes a simple but important
modification is introduced which transforms the circular conception into a spiral—ever on a rising incline, because time enters
the picture as an inescapable element. In this plan too, there is a
system of returns to points resembling the earlier positions. In the
age of reason, in the 18th Century, quite naturally, the idea dawned
that history could describe a course of continuous more or less
uninterrupted progress. It was Professor J. B. Bury who called
attention to the *Observations on the Continuous Progress of Universal Reason* which the Abbé de Saint-Pierre published in 1737.
That was the first time, Bury tells us, that "the vista of an immensely long progressive life" was placed "in front of humanity."
But it was far from the last. In the past century, both in Europe
and in America, almost everyone was immersed in ideas originating in the doctrine of evolution. We were persuaded that civilization is a continuous process, passing onward from stage to stage,
losing nothing, every discovery and every conception being added
to all the preceding ones with the hope that, whatever the current
vicissitudes, we were becoming better and better. We were so
convinced that this was so we ceased even to trouble to inquire
whether we might not be mistaken. We were convinced. We
went so far as to omit teaching the history of the struggle for the
attainment of freedom. We took it for granted. We needed no
further persuasion that we were in fact becoming better and
better. I remember, as a small boy, to have been vastly comforted
because I heard my father confide to one of his friends that he
thought on the whole the world was getting better. We were
forgetting to ask, "Better than what?" or "Better toward what
end?" Quite obviously toward what end might make a difference;

better at an insight into the nature of God; or better in a knowledge of the liberal arts; or better in the use of the materials which the operation of the scientific process puts into our hands. We should be asking, "Better than what?" Better than a civilized Athenian of the 4th Century? We are in no doubt now whether the successors of the Greeks, in the German woods, say in the 4th Century of this era, were superior to their Greek predecessors. We no longer agree with Rousseau. The Golden Age, even if it does not lie ahead, certainly does not lie behind us.

What else can all of this mean than that the conception, civilization, is not a definitive arrangement, cut to a predetermined pattern, valid for all time, to be taken down from the shelf of history, to be fitted together, to be applied and lived whenever we choose to live it. There is nothing it seems that can, offhand, be called civilization, to be gained or lost, in some arbitrary way. It is more likely that a civilization is life in being, constantly becoming, and ultimately forming a structure with characteristic local features. The pattern arises under circumstances into the conditioning of which we need not now inquire, except that we know that its being our own, made by us and suiting our tastes and our nature, decides us in our loyalty to it. In the United States we have relatively little difficulty in identifying its elements. There were Greek elements and Roman elements. There is a powerful element derived from 17th Century England, especially the scene of religious, political and economic wars, inhospitable to persons of dissident religious faiths. Dissenters, many of them, emigrated, preferring life on an untrammeled and politically free continent, by good fortune recently discovered and opened for settlement. Out of that episode grew tolerance. The 18th Century contributed still another element. Facts and theories of politics and economics developed in a direction to make possible a fresh choice to those to whom the exercise of free will and the opportunity for free choice had become not only congenial but necessary. When all of this had been assimilated, more or less, what we call our civilization started off in a series of revolutions both here and abroad. Fresh choices were made. Men asserted opposition to ways of life habitual to Europe but becoming uncongenial. They initiated their new governments with declarations in which the words life, liberty and the pursuit of happiness appeared; or their French equivalent liberty, equality and fraternity. The former was our Declaration of Independence. Then came the first amendments to our Constitution. We now know such pronouncements as bills of rights. They declare the right and the wisdom of withdrawal from ancient and outworn ways and the adoption of new ones—not wholly new as those who recall the Annapolis and other spirited and learned debates of that day remember. They established the framework within which the first century and a half of the history of the United States evolved. The choices, the precise forms, that were offered to the citizens of the late 18th Century and the early 19th, were not simple, even if they were not new. Plutocracy, oligarchy, democracy, even monarchy were advocated and carefully examined as the Jefferson-Hamilton controversies and the papers in the Federalist amply demonstrate. As the century wore on, the interests of industry as against those of agriculture became intensified and were ever more fiercely asserted until there was no escape from or, to put the issue from the point of view I am urging, there remained no other *choice* except civil war. It is an important speculation whether an act like the Wages and Hours Bill, if enacted in the year 1850, might not have provided a technique in the domain of reason for avoiding that conflict. We have chosen now to enact that Bill with the ultimate, perhaps unexpressed intention, of forestalling a comparable controversy and of solving an issue which involves the economic future of the country. What it is important to understand is that within the framework of our basic beliefs, reason and, therefore, choice can enter into our decisions. The vehicles are education, the ballot, legislation, administration, and the courts.

Meanwhile industrial organization instead of remaining simple has become ever more complex. From being small it has become great, from having grown powerful, it came in the time of Theodore Roosevelt, to dominate government. Against this power, the natural reaction has been, through organization, increase in counter power of workers and smaller people on farms and in towns. Government itself has developed techniques to meet these issues until it has become necessary to look forward to a time when choice is removed from the simple direct volition of the many, the individual citizens, to a concentration of their wishes expressed through their own large and powerful organizations.

Because these issues are great they do not become less grave. They are grave because they are still in the region where decision is possible or where we must behave as if this were still the case. How they are decided affects the well-being of every citizen. To retreat, under these circumstances, from the effort at understanding the argument through becoming acquainted with the relevant factors involved in a situation which is intricate but not too intricate to be understood, is to sell one's birthright. The issues are grave, but they need not be beyond, indeed I think they can be brought within, the comprehension of the average citizen. He must take part in the debate, learning the nature of the issues. If he neglects engaging in it, he contributes conceivably to his own undoing. He must not complain if advocates of a program or of a solution place their views before him in a form calculated to obscure his vision, in order to win his approval. We need to become fully instructed in the form of debate. We need to learn the *meaning* of the arguments that are used. We need to inquire about the consequences of the possible decisions. Greek sophists have explained what an advocate in a debate must plead and how an opponent must meet his attack. The facts must become known. The arguments of both sides must insist on whether a statement based on the facts is probable. But to be vigilant about the form of the debate is not enough. More, much more is needed. Among the things that men say, wheat must be separated from chaff. We must be prepared to understand the meaning of plans and of arguments. If you are told a thing is "good," you must ask "good for what?" If you are told the assertion of individual rights leads to fascism, you must be very certain what the exercise of individual rights implies, you must know precisely what this particular advocate means by fascism, whether it is rule by the few or rule by the many, and if by the few, whether they be rich or poor and in whose interest they wish to rule, in yours or in theirs. You must be certain concerning your interests. You must know whether the two are identical. If you are told rule must be exercised for the good of the nation, you are entitled to ask what is meant by the nation and what role you play within its structure. If you are invited to wage war, your thinking and your training should have prepared you to inquire to what end that war is to be waged. Is it to ward off an enemy, or to capture another people to enslave them, or to capture a market; is it to defend the exercise of your beliefs or to impose your belief on other people? Designing men attempt to confuse our counsels. But we can be certain of this, unless we have a plan of life, unless we have decided on our objective, unless we understand how our choice is likely to operate, unless we perceive as clearly as may be, whether a procedure will accomplish our aim, wariness and further inquiry are necessary. We have for example, for very good and sufficient reason, come to believe we wish the way of our lives to be the ways of freedom. We have come to rest our faith in the belief that the best way to maintain freedom for individuals is by the use of the ballot, by the organization of great political parties. We may have perceived that a multiplicity of parties, though certain ends are served, such as a more exact expression on the part of a few of their desires, has worked abroad in such a way as to confuse the presentation and deliberations of major issues, and has worked in the end to the undoing of orderly democratic procedure and of the attainment of desirable democratic ends. Competent critics declare that the techniques of proportional representation, good as it may be for some purposes, worked in Germany under the Weimar Constitution, in so far as an administrative instrument can be regarded as contributing to the sequel, to the destruction of the German Republic. Professor Hermens of the Catholic University of America [2] has written powerfully in advocacy of this belief. The use of reason requires an exploration of such an issue. If we are told proportional representation is good, we must ask, let me repeat, "good for what?" If we are told it is good because through its use we can destroy the republic, we may think twice before, in an unguarded manner, we introduce it into the national procedure.

[2] Now at Notre Dame University.

It may be necessary to decide whether, in order to secure a desideratum, the price exacted is not placed too high.

And so constituting this civilization there are, it appears, a multiplicity of elements, the accumulations or the deposits of time. In the very language of that civilization may be found a guide to the many peoples who have contributed to its form. Greek, Roman, Hebrew and Arabic are scattered thickly through almost every extended utterance. And so also are ideas, of God, of marriage, of law, of goodness, of tolerance, of freedom, whether of speech, of press, or assembly; of the right of every man to the benefits of the Bill of Rights; of the value of education, to Jefferson most important perhaps of all; of justice, and of how to attain it. Taken in the large, recognizable threads run through its texture and give it cohesion and consistence. In order that the scheme shall work, one without the other may turn out to be impracticable or, perhaps, impossible. Certain ones the organizers of the Nation chose to write into our Constitution. What has clustered legitimately about it, as its irreducible essence, we in this society call our civilization.

Even so, many men would say, "This is not enough; that is not all." Civilization is something more. What they think should be added is what we perceive as the physical appearance of our world—the way we build our houses, how these are assembled in villages, towns and cities, the fact that we transport our bodies and our goods frequently and rapidly from place to place in trains and in automobiles and in the air. What difference that alone makes will be made dramatically plain on recalling Henry Adams's eloquent description of the state of communication in the United States in the year 1800. Other elements in the appearance, perhaps the surface appearances of our lives, must include electricity and the all but unimaginable uses to which that has been put by applied science and technology. In any modern mechanized farm, if two copper wires were to break, heat would cease to be generated in houses heated with oil-burning furnaces; food would not be cooked because of dependence on electric ranges; at night houses would remain in darkness; if water were pumped with a motor it would be necessary to do without it—without heat, light, cooking, water, ice—all dependent on two copper wires, the playthings of the elements. I need not recapitulate the innumerable ways in which discovery, invention, manufacture of foods, clothing, furniture, have transformed every aspect of our lives. Beside ideas, customs, and behavior, these contributions of pure science and applied science have shaped our existence. All together—food, shelter, clothing, beliefs, and conduct are inextricably interwoven. They fit each other as pebbles come to be faceted by constant intimacy, by friction, by wearing away, by mutual adaptation.

Now these are not the elements which every civilization exhibits. This scheme may have cohesion, may be consistent, and its elements may appear to be indissolubly assembled. But it is only one of the forms with which we are familiar even in our day. It is not an inalienable possession—this civilization of ours. We may lose it. Some say we should thereby recapture our own soul. But if we lose it, must we lose it in whole or can it be abandoned in part—can we decide to modify it by casting out spurious elements, by limiting the exercise of harmful mechanical or scientific processes, by modifying the law or the Constitution? What it is essential to comprehend is that our civilization has a shape, that no matter what the external, no matter what the environmental compulsions, we, consciously and unconsciously both, gave it that shape—and in its essence gave it that shape in our ancient history, in the 18th and again in the 19th Centuries, undoubtedly in certain of its elements from choice, after due reflection and extended debate. We made it, and so it can be unmade. If we are driven to undertake to unmake it, we assume a heavy responsibility. Being man made, in large measure it must be man secured. If eternal vigilance is the price of liberty, it is at least as relevant now, as ever it was, to utter this warning.

Civilizations can have, as is abundantly clear, many complexions. If a civilization is not quite a garment that can willfully be put off, corresponding more or less intimately to the genius of the society that made it and having appropriateness to its time and place, the society which has evolved it or which has adopted it and to which it is appropriate has, nevertheless, given to it something individual. In a general way, the English (and the French

before Vichy), live under dispensations in many respects similar
to our own and yet no one would regard the ways of life of these
three communities (they may properly be termed societies) as
being identical. The difference is the measure of their individuality
and represents the extent to which it is possible to employ the
word "society." The factors involved in establishing the differences depend without doubt on the influence of geography; but
beside geography, history plays its own conspicuous role. In a sense,
a society documents its individuality in the selection or the rejec-
tion of elements of contemporary novelty; it takes what suits it—
it rejects the rest.

Now a society, being a collection of human beings, differs from
a civilization in the assemblage of manners and customs which
that society manifests. A society is that group, originating in a
large variety of ways, which manifests those choices as to purpose,
function, and law to which I have already referred. Our own
society has deliberately chosen and keeps on choosing as its leaders,
Moses and Christ, Plato and Aristotle; Dante and Shakespeare,
Shelley and Wordsworth; Galilei and Harvey; Copernicus and
Lavoisier; Pasteur and Lister, Faraday and Maxwell and Gibbs;
Volta and Edison, Morse and Marconi; Bach and Beethoven,
Brahms and Wagner, Giotto, Rembrandt and Michelangelo;
Samuel Adams and Patrick Henry; Washington and Jefferson;
Madison and Lincoln. What these men thought and did is our
civilization. Not so long ago France, when it was offered a single
choice, chose Pasteur. Each society does in this way choose its
laws and its heroes. And by their choices are they known.

Our society, while passing through the crucible of its birth,
attained its form through mature deliberation and the sufferings
of two wars. The debates before the War of the Revolution, before the adoption of the Constitution, before the Civil War are,
as anyone familiar with them knows, as fine a flowering of the
function of reason in exploring ways of corporate existence as is
to be found in political literature. If ever reason was adopted as
a guide to conduct, and if ever reason prevailed in the analysis of
a complex social context, it did so here. Its great achievement is

that the scheme has worked. From the results of that enterprise retreat is now unthinkable.

A few short years ago the question of retreat was scarcely raised in these United States. More recently on two fronts, on the front of political science and on the front of natural science, defeatist voices have been raised. The suggestion is made that in some manner, not clearly understood, the operations of reason have somehow mystically failed. Men begin to forget that in the 18th Century, when escape from the ancient regime was being planned, the fate of the common man was at least as much debated as it is now and that then, not for the first time, examination of his problems in the light first of sympathetic understanding and then of reason was successfully undertaken. Ever since, in these 150 years, life has been lived under the dispensation then formulated. All this seems in process of being too easily forgotten, of being too lightly brushed aside. We are told democracy is facing failure (1) partly because we cannot control the results of the operation of science, and (2) partly because in the march of economic organization we lack the insight and the power to master our destiny. Being man made in its building, no doubt we can unmake what has been so elaborately constructed.

But why? There is general agreement that what has been achieved has not been equaled either in the standard of general living, in the opportunity for further development, or in the degree, obviously not yet superlative, of satisfactoriness in our intellectual and spiritual lives. How if, in our democratic faith, the method of reason has had this measure of constructive achievement to its credit, can the conclusion be drawn that reason is bankrupt? Study, deep study, is on the march. In the various offices of the League of Nations, in the explorations of the Independent Labour Office, in the Commissions of President Hoover, in the investigations of Committees of the Congress, in Great Britain through reports of Royal Commissions, as frank, as fearless, as intelligent efforts to solve social problems in an incredibly complex economic background, have been undertaken as ever in the rough adjustments of Western societies.

And in science, how is retreat possible? The progress onward of science can be likened to the movement of a train of freight cars. Articles of value have for centuries been accepted as cargo. The pressure pump, the magnetic compass, the telescope have all been regarded as articles of value. So have the telegraph, the telephone, the radio, the railways, genetics, bacteria and physiology; rayon, cellulose, electric light and the products of power engineering. Reason, the same reason, has been at work when the use of these agencies turns out to be beneficent as when it has been turned to uses hostile and deadly. When the attempt is made, as has recently been done, to find ways of deflecting discoveries and inventions away from evil uses, it becomes a social responsibility of the first order to gain correct insights into what doing this means. Otherwise there can be no correct decisions.

There is beyond doubt, the possibility of disaster through the misuse of discovery. Scientists, as has been pointed out, are integral parts of our society. They carry the burden for getting on with the business of accumulating natural knowledge. They do so in large part as social agents, but in part also as citizens. In the interest of the national safety they may omit no act likely to serve the interests of their group. In the interest of national comfort they are not likely to do so. But political arrangement intra- or international is not their primary function. That function is the responsibility of politicians and statesmen. Scientists can go no further, I think, than to point out the consequences of their discoveries. How to use them humanely is not their concern further than it is that of other citizens. Is it not unreasonable to hold them responsible for accomplishing that which they are told off by the rest of society, their ultimate employers, to devise—for good or evil? Power of decision, in the end, does not rest in their hands. Before interfering with the scientific process, before deciding which of its contributions is harmful, it behooves us to explore the workings of so complex a mechanism, remembering the assumption that we are somehow in control of our destiny. What do we stop, if we stop scientific research?

And by the same token what do we find, if we examine social behavior? It is a subject, the latter, which Shaw analyzed to

good purpose in *Arms and the Man.* There is no way decently
in which to justify man's inhumanity to man. To curb it, law, in
the form of the *Decalogue,* has appeared among us; and persuasion in that of the *Sermon on the Mount,* their predecessors and
successors through all time. The reign of conscious effort has, as
time goes, been brief—not so brief but that we are already conscious of evil and are setting in motion the agencies of ameliora-
tion. To curb seems infinitely preferable to destroying; to correct
and modify, as functions of reason, to dispensing with reason. The
will to goodness is strong—stronger, I believe than is often
recognized and stronger as I think than ever before. The view
is general that the same degree of success in social control has not
been attained that is so apparent in the control of nature—success
of natural science as opposed to social and political science. That
judgment is often accepted as self-apparent. But it must be clear
that we do not control nature. What we control are a few forces
of nature—not the tides, not the winds, not the movement of
the crust of the earth. We are a little deceived by our words. In
appraising the difference between natural and political science, is
it captious to ask for the evidence? To be certain that it is correct,
a yardstick is wanted. But where is that yardstick to be found?
To be able to measure these two advancing fronts, social and
scientific, would be desirable had we proper instruments. Obviously the better a yardstick is made to measure the one, the less
likely is its success in measuring the other. Measuring is a function of the thing that is to be measured. Yardsticks are made to
measure yards. The mind of man has been powerfully concerned
with both fronts. It seems unwise to destroy one because we suspect,
correctly or incorrectly, we cannot manage the other—unwise to
restrain science until we learn how to restrain men. There is in
point of fact social control—in large measure. There is the force
of public opinion; orderliness without omnipresent police; control
by means of a simple white line drawn down the middle of the
road. And in a larger sphere has it not been justly observed that

   Peace to the world from ports without a gun

has turned out to be a possibility?

Suppose we decide not to destroy science but to curb it. But how? The belief is widespread that there are two kinds of science, disinterested science and purposeful science. We should without doubt not oppose advance in the disinterested variety. How is this end to be achieved? How has science been made? Nothing affected the thought of the 17th and 18th Centuries like the discovery of the law of gravitation and the laws of motion. On no subject has Voltaire been more eloquent. Nothing seemed more innocent. But if the analysis of Hessen is correct, Galilei's interest, and Newton's, were derived in large part from concern with military affairs, with metals and forces. Science like that grows, as men would now say, out of sin—if war is sin. And to the extent that these laws are the operating cornerstones of all the science that has come afterward, these discoveries have issued again—in sin. All our crimes, all our mechanical civilization, have issued from these innocent calculations. On a lesser level, as much can no doubt be said of every other first-rate scientific speculation. The gas laws are not unrelated to explosion nor the facts of anthropology to misconceptions of race. Astronomy and explosives, aeronautics and bombing are not far apart.

It is conceivable that protection can be found against misuse. Do we not paint red the wagons that carry explosives? And yet such protection is directed not against the primary activity of research, applied to the analysis of natural phenomena, but to derivatives in positions at the 2nd or 3rd or 4th remove. In spite of such reflections I prefer not to take the defeatist position, not to restrain the urge to discovery. Better management will come, not with applying less reason but with the exercise of more, not with ignoring our problems but with an ever greater effort to solve them.

This society, at all events, is dedicated to the notion that this civilization, deeply rooted in regard for the common man, developed by experience and achieved through reason operating as social and scientific thought, shall advance to the greater good of man and to the realization of a greater measure of human contentment.

On Retiring

SOME time since, Professor Perry, a man of learning and of great natural charm, seeing the way the world was going, entered with pathos and fortitude a "Plea for an Age Movement." [1] It was a happy conception and the intervention timely, though there were those who thought it was already overdue. We elders were being beset by un-understanding, because still emotionally underdeveloped, foes. Naturally they meant us no harm, but they were not on our side of the divide. How could they know on theirs, what we felt and thought? We had not begun to fight.

This is not a simple problem. Had I Professor Perry's gift I should try to suggest a solution as enticingly satisfactory, at first glance anyway, as his in the case of King David and King Solomon. So that there be no misunderstanding, let me repeat his thesis for you. He took it from James Ball Naylor.

> King David and King Solomon
>   Led merry, merry lives,
> With many, many lady friends
>   And many, many wives;
> But when old age crept over them—
>   With many, many qualms,
> King Solomon wrote the Proverbs
>   And King David wrote the Psalms.

Now that was all right for King David and King Solomon—for them to write the Psalms and the Proverbs. In any case they did what they pleased. They did not *have* to retire. But who wants to write Psalms and Proverbs? In the first place, they have been written. And then, despite the scribe, that proposal presents no pattern of life in this modern world.

[1] *Plea for an Age Movement*, New York, 1942.

32

It seems, all over again, that there is no teacher but experience. How is a man of 44 to guess the worth of his elders? How can he know, unless he had experienced what Confucius discovered when he reached the top of Tai Shan and, looking down on the Kingdom of Liu, found that the land he had left behind was very inconsiderable?

The trouble is that we have been the architects of our own undoing. We have not published forth what we still can do. So, not having declared our value, there seemed to be only one solution of our problem: Off with our heads. It works very well too. Once a man's head is off, his personal problem is solved. And because he says nothing—utters no word of protest and none of illumination, the obvious and uncontradicted conclusion is, he has nothing to say. That makes everything much easier. I do not disagree. But about King David and King Solomon—as a natural scientist of sorts, I should like to have known more of the events that intervened between the ribaldry of the early lives of these gentry and of the evolution of their later piety. Perhaps, if we did, we should find that their solutions were undoubtedly possible for them. But for us—Proverbs, "Yes," but Psalms, "No." In any case the whole of this evolution is a little improbable. We should prefer, should we not, a little more orderliness than a direct passage from merry lives and many wives and lady friends —over to the Proverbs and the Psalms.

I should like to persuade you to approach this future of ours in a more reflective fashion, as befits scholars and men of science. Much of our trouble has come from having had a bad press. I see nothing lovely in the lives of Noah or Methuselah. Socrates did not do badly—perhaps later on, had he not worried his fellow-townsmen to his own undoing, he would have become more mellow and maybe even comprehensible. In my opinion, Cicero has been almost dead weight. It would have been much better if he had not written a sententious and pompous piece, to remind everyone who came after him that men can be dull, and older men— dull, as it were, by profession. Our motto, I say, should be: "Up and coming—business as usual."

One of the most pessimistic of reporters was a man named

Shakespeare. Aside from the lugubrious misinformation he put into the mouth of that melancholy Jaques, he made inaccurate calculations about the ages of man. His divisions I suspect are wrong and the sixth picture, of "the lean and slipper'd pantaloon" and the seventh, "last scene of all . . . (of) second childishness and mere oblivion," I am certain have been harmful, hurtful and deplorable fictions.

Most recent of all is that quasi-divinity of ours, Dr. Osler. What he said made a great furor at the time (February 22, 1905) and ruined what chances might have been ours. He referred nostalgically to Anthony Trollope's "plot (that) hinges upon the admirable scheme of a college into which at sixty men retired for a year of contemplation before a peaceful departure by chloroform." Naturally no one remembers his mitigating clause: "I have become a little dubious, as my own time is getting so short." But he said something else too, for which much shall be forgiven him. I will keep that for an appropriate place later on.

No; this is not the right line. In this brave new world of ours, we must be modern. We must demonstrate who we are—that we are men with honorable pasts, full of the wisdom of experience, and full of new inescapable notions of how this world is to be managed. And there is plenty of evidence to encourage us that we do right, when we propose to leave the doldrums behind.

But first, everybody must be made aware that we are not a race whom the Reaper has all but annihilated. That was true once upon a time. Things are very different now. I can show that—some of it anyway—from statistics. Take the women. Unhappily just statistical women. Before the fifteen-hundreds, there is not much information. Of those who survived the first fifteen years, only half (50 per cent) reached 50 years and less than a tenth (9 per cent) reached 75. The 2787 women who constitute this story flourished in the best circles, in fact among the ruling families of Europe. These pampered darlings of privilege had the best food, the best houses, the best personal hygiene, the best medical care that were available. And besides they were not worked to death.

Times change. Nowadays, women wear scarcely enough to

keep them warm, not from choice, A. V. Hill to the contrary notwithstanding. They smoke, they drink, they flock, I hope less often to their physicians than to beauticians. But the astonishing thing is that now, not a half but actually more than four-fifths (87 per cent) attain 50; and not one-tenth (9 per cent) but almost six-tenths (57 per cent) reach 75. They have come to do better—by more than 600 per cent.

Women have often achieved the better things of life. They should—and so, in this business of living long, have outstripped the men. They still do. About the same number (86.6 per cent) of men get to be 50, but when it comes to 75, men muster only 35.3 per cent against the women's 57—22 per cent less. But in a way that may be the better luck.

That brings us face to face with our great dilemma. The world was unprepared for so many of us. Methuselah is no longer to be taken with a grain of mythological salt. He is here and he is a whole army. He literally teems. But more threatening still, he is *no* pantaloon. That is where Shakespeare did us the great injury declaring that in the sixth age, we did nothing. Actually we pull a strong and steady oar, and probably we always did.

Take Cervantes. He managed the second part of *Don Quixote* when he was 68. Or take Goethe; he published the First Part of *Faust* at 59. The Second Part came out the year after his death at 83. Or Henry James who entered his great *Major Phase*, we are now learning, between 60 and 73.

If that world does not interest you, take this one. Our Secretary of War [2] is 77. The Chief of the General Staff [3] is 64. General MacArthur is 65. Admiral Leahy is 69. Admiral King is 66. Admiral Hepburn is 67. Admiral Horne is 65. General Knudsen is 65. May I mention the not quite harmless Field Marshal v. Rundstedt? [4] He is 69.

All these men were officially dead. For our good they had to be revived—by Act of Congress. How good that chloroform was not written as an optional into the law. The uniformitarians might then sooner or later have wanted to make its use obligatory.

[2] Henry L. Stimson.
[3] George C. Marshall.

[4] This essay was contemporary with the Battle of the Bulge, 1944.

Or if you don't like that world either, take this one. Darwin
published his *Origins* at 50 and his *Descent of Man* at 62. Crookes
invented the radiometer at 63. Pasteur did the first inoculation
at 63 and kept on going until he was 75. Harvey published his
De Motu Cordis at 50 and his *De Generatione* at 73. In the
latter he discovered to us that *omnis vivum* originated *ex ovo*. No
mean discovery either—at 73.

Or if you are dissatisfied with these worlds, take this one. The
Justices and Judges of the United States used to serve during
good behavior. Then, in 1869, this lumbering but flexible government of ours changed the rules. After ten years of service, you
could if you chose retire at 70. There have been 83 Justices
altogether. Forty-five served after 65—more than half (54.2 per
cent). I recall Justice Holmes's saying that in a world of amusement, to write an opinion, perhaps a minority opinion, at 91 is also
an amusement. And no one doubted he did it very well. For more
than twenty-five years after the official academic age of death, he
was still counted among the great and compelling and shining
examples of professional and philosophical competence. The quality
of the opinions of many another of them encourages a belief in this
scheme and suggests the pitiful injury that would be done if they
were forced to retire.

Let me repeat. We took the world by surprise, because of our
great and increasing numbers. Suddenly it was discovered we
clogged the machine. No one knew what to do. The Autocrat
said once, at the Breakfast Table, that "if a man were to be
burned in any of our cities tomorrow for heresy, there would be
found a master of ceremonies who knew just how many faggots
were necessary, and the best way of arranging the whole matter."
This is called *argumentum ad ignem*. So, what more natural than
that in our case someone thought of the method of the Queen
of Hearts.

"A cat may look at a king," said Alice. "I've read that in some
book but I don't remember where."

"Well, it must be removed," said the King very decidedly, and he
called to the Queen, who was passing at the moment, "My dear! I
wish you would have this cat removed!"

The Queen had only one way of settling all difficulties, great or small. "Off with his head!" she said, without even looking round.

It is said to be a painless method. Many of us do not even mind. Others are converting pain into joy. And the dear administrators are thinking of making still other and novel provisions for us. They are going to teach the poor old things how to play. Their declining days are to be cheered and lightened. One of the old *Fables for the Frivolous* has been driven home. Should we not stop laying for the innocent geese (ganders, of course), just because they have been laying for us? If younger men and women are clamoring for their posts and perhaps also their salaries, can we not do better than to insist upon their going? Of course the selection of the time of departure may be postponed too long. They may become too disspirited to learn new games. But there is a way out. You remember how Father William prepared himself:

> "You are old, Father William," the young man said,
>   "And your hair has become very white;
> And yet you incessantly stand on your head—
>   Do you think, at your age, it is right?"
>
> "In my youth," Father William replied to his son,
>   "I feared it might injure the brain;
> But, now that I'm perfectly sure I have none,
>   Why, I do it again and again."

So now there are to be kindergartens for the middle-aged, to learn how to play when old. Of course they could go on using their brains—perhaps even powerfully. But maybe there is no need in an active world—or is there not? Perhaps "Yes," if we could be persuaded that experience, and plans that grow out of experience, had value.

It would be only fair to look into the mind of the academic Queen of Hearts. Why has she chosen an arbitrary age for decapitation? She must have studied the business profoundly and wisely perhaps and sympathetically. She must have looked into what men can do at 50 and 60 and 70. Does she really know whether cutting off heads really doesn't hurt? Has she inquired

into whether she really has no use for older statesmen? Is the
kingdom of Academe so knowingly and so fruitfully governed
that she can afford to thrust the tried and the true into outer
limbo? The usual alibi is that uniform cutting off of heads is
fairer than bothering to go to a court of justice about every individual's fate. " 'Off with his head,' without even looking round."
It's the only way of settling all difficulties, great and small. It is
more humane that the just and the unjust should suffer alike.

But why go in for suffering? Why routineer? Why not explore a little further? Why not learn from the young—about
vocational guidance for the old? This may not be much of a
problem after all.

Clearly this is no laughing matter. A first solution was not
beyond the reach of philanthropists with warm hearts. That accounts for Mr. Pritchett's bright hopes and Mr. Carnegie's generosity. At first everything seemed easy and practicable. But our
friends miscalculated. We multiplied too rapidly and kept on
multiplying.

I know how alive our experts are to the emotional and other
imponderables in this delicate situation. They know the actuarial
problems. Will not the cost be prohibitive? No doubt it can be
heavy, but perhaps not too heavy when you reckon in the great
service that can be rendered and would be, by experienced and
willing men. If there are relatively *few* who have *nothing* to offer
—well, then the cost may be well worth bearing. The morale of
a society, we are learning, has saving value. And morale is the
higher when it lives in hope rather than in depression and fear.
Delicacy suggests first and foremost, I think, the elimination of
the pecuniary hurdle. Money curdles so much and so often, the
sweet milk of human organization. What actually happens is
that powerless individuals become the *noblesse* of the famous
mot, rather than the strong institutions. Unfortunately they are
asked both to bear the cost and to exercise the *oblige* term of
that same *mot.*

I call Osler to witness, the one who did us so poor a turn. He
actually recommended "The teacher's life should have three periods, study until twenty-five, investigation until forty, profession

until sixty, at which age I would have him retired on a double allowance." Now, say I, if you are going to appeal to authority here is where Osler is our proper man.

Let me go back to the Supreme Court. After the new rule of 1869, money fortunately played no role in deciding whether Justices are to serve or to retire. At 70, after ten years of service, they may go; but their salaries go on undiminished until the final roll call. That rule provides an excellent experiment. No one stays after 70, having served ten years—for money. The poll stands this way: Between the time of Chief Justice Marshall (1801) and the adoption of the new retiring rule, the eleven who reached 70 all served on. Afterwards, of 27 eligibles, only one retired. Clearly salary which continued in any event can have played no role in the decision of a Justice either to stay or to go. Naturally everybody did not die in harness. Before 1869, only one retired (at 82). After 1869, 17 did—only 4 before 75. Has it been worth it? How do we measure opinion? Take these ten names after the rule. There were Bradley, Brandeis, Brown, Field, Fuller, Holmes, Miller, Taft, Van Devanter, White—would their going not have been a loss?

Soldiering in this context has no meaning. Whoever has read the correspondence between Justice Holmes and Sir Frederick Pollock must be impressed with the volume of work that Holmes delighted to achieve even at 90. Young men work no harder. Holmes groaned cheerfully. Would any man carry such a burden unless he wanted to! A Justice need do so on no other count.

Naturally there are many susceptibilities to safeguard. To let one man go, being no longer wanted, not having attained proper distinction or having failed to advance his science or not having endeared himself to his colleagues— while inviting his brother to continue has little humane to recommend it. But, we are told, this uniform system is in essence the most humane. You are tempted to object that it might be, if it were really carried out. But you discover it is not fair even if it were—either to the scholars or to society—unfair to the scholars, some of whom wish to stay and should; while others wish to go and may without damage; and unfair to society which can still make good use of them. We came near just now of being deprived of almost the whole higher command of our military establishment. And yet, if you object, you are told: "Oh, yes! We know. Some do stay while others go. Between ourselves we must tell you we are not so unintelligent as to treat everybody alike." Well, you give it up. You wonder at a system that knows how to be fair because it does treat everybody alike and claims to be fairer still because it doesn't.

In short the misfortune of making distinctions is not avoided now. It is a fact that many scholars would welcome a chance to choose new occupations or to get at old ones from new angles. A librarian may wish to turn historian, and a novelist a biographer; or a mathematician, a philosopher; and a physician, an etcher. Are there not many men in whom two strains travel along side by side? One like the serpent strain in Elsie Venner, may die out, but the other, the long overshadowed human one, unlike the snake in Elsie, at last can go on to new, released and vigorous life. That would be like a glorified vacation—to do all the things for which in a busy life there has been no time. Now you can enjoy your best thoughts and communicate them.

Of course, many men, everywhere, have no other craving than to go on. Nowadays they are to be encountered all over the place accepting, as it were, post-prandial positions. They represent the return of that appealing creature—the wandering scholar. Now he is the wandering Emeritus. His lot is a little better now. He used to be desperately poor. He wanders still, but fortunately on half-pay, at least. Could there not be created new positions, called something else than Emeritus—*regular* positions, freer maybe of former distasteful routines or unwanted responsibility, *new* positions that would provide more elbow room and broader scope? These would be positions of promotion or of honor—not giving the impression of discard. They would provide the opportunity for making graceful gestures instead of contriving unhappy dismissals and the misfortune of avoidable bitterness. And places, no minor consideration, would more systematically be made for justly impatient younger scholars. The very notion I am suggesting would be foolish if there were not, as now, dissatisfaction abroad.

What is objectionable now is the argument, on some ground of no greater human significance than a workable administrative device, that one's work is done. For serious men it is in truth, as Justice Holmes said in his radio address, *never done.*

If I go on in this way there will be complaint; benevolence will be offended. We shall hear: "What do the *vieillards* expect? Indefinite tenure? Have they not been encouraged and sustained the major part of their lives? Have they not chosen their Procrustean beds—not made their bargain with Fate and Fortune?" There is a point here. Consider for a moment the situation of the great and the rich and the powerful. They too have made their choice. They have cast their nets into the waters. They keep hauling in loaves and fishes. Theirs are teeming waters, counted on to be productive. But how much sounder they, than the improvident scholar who courts only opportunity to understand and to know, to enjoy the play of his mind and to serve. If perchance wealth and power cling for a while, perchance even for a generation or two, while the gifts and graces of the scholar's spirit have not that enduring advantage, would they not be foolish in Calverley's idiom if they made of themselves something else when God made of them something so fortunate? An improvident academic race must take warning. If they follow the pleasures of the mind rather than the wisdom of the body, who else but themselves will pay the price? In this social system it is the social values of that system which are at stake. In the current dispensation there is no other way unless somehow we recast our values and then somehow rewrite, *He who pays the piper can call the tune.*

Have you expected me to describe the dimming of a man's eyes and the aging of his brain; to speak about his arteries and his heart, about his kidneys and his bones? I have not done so because they are only parts of a man. You cannot show whether he is better or worse by demonstrating that his organs are not up to snuff. You must take him as he is—all in all—a going concern. I have been asking instead: Is he going, or still going, or going wrong, or going ahead? In truth I find that no two are going alike and that every somebody is going his own separate way.

The Influence of Modern Science on Painting and Sculpture

THE INFLUENCE of modern science on painting and sculpture can mean many things, for the 19th Century itself presented not a single but a variety of antithetical moods. What was left of the revolution or revolutions, what the temper was of Victorianism, what Darwin, Marx, Clerk Maxwell, Willard Gibbs, Helmholtz, Faraday and Sigmund Freud contributed to the sum of the effects constitute a complex which requires a wide variety of treatment. Nor should there be omitted from the account the kind of science represented by the school of exact historians, Mommsen, Grote, Acton, Maitland, Turner and Haskins. Here are varieties of influence, all illustrating that positive, factual, rational, evolving train of intellectual background against which painting and sculpture may be observed and their meaning estimated. It would be an error to view the progress of effort in the Century as emerging from a source designated a cause and spreading out into a series of happenings to be regarded as its effects.

The facts would be more nearly represented if there could be identification of those motives which, forming a complex climate of opinion, permeated all thought and subsequently, of course, all feeling and dominated finally the vast variety of activities which characterized these one hundred or more years. Beyond everything it would be an error to disregard the continuum which stretched back to the Renaissance and the Reformation and the rebirth of scientific learning. That event can be identified as having occurred in the 16th Century though more likely it had its origin further back in the 13th. To link the contributions of the 19th to periods anteceding the 18th is distinctly rewarding but unnecessary. There it is imperative to discern the beginnings of the revolution in industry and the temper of the revolution, both, together with science, playing significant, determining roles in time ahead.

It would be a further error not to think of these strains as mutually interwoven, the warp and woof of a common life. The complexion of life, somehow is always a whole—in our own you cannot disregard plumbing, flying, automobiles, short skirts, the movies, unemployment, the struggle for freedom, the theory of relativity, skyscrapers. They are part and parcel of our mental horizon and daily experience. To omit one would do excessive violence to the picture of daily living which is evoked when the suggestion of what a day contains receives reference.

The need for infinite attention to many things in detail, to vast developments in mechanization, to gadgets, to the necessity that things must work has fastened attention to reality, of a sort that has made it incumbent on us to identify parts and shapes and the movements of machines—to make us insist on exact description in ways which are new. In another age, Degas would have cared less about the exact movements of dancers or of ways of running of race horses.

The unity of life is altogether worth insisting upon. It tends to dispel the notion that one thing proceeds from some other isolated thing rather than as the result of everything, taken together, that goes on in one's conscious and subconscious being. If life progresses on a wide front and throws out pseudopods in this or that direction, there exist behind that front the innumerable forces, great and small of which the whole of our being is informed. In what I have been saying I have wished to suggest that in using the word "influence," what is intended is not some simple relation of cause and effect but a mass impact of the life and interests of a society on the minds of those, artists and scientists, who are moved to give expression, each one in an idiom peculiar to himself, to something that moves the rest of us also, in ways equally appropriate. For all of us are bound together having our motivating power in an identical matrix of thought, action, and emotion. The point then would be that, without in the least relying upon something to be interpreted in a mystical sense, there is a way of feeling the nature of one's world, of wishing to share one's experience of it, such that being temperamentally oneself, one gives utterance, because one must, in that medium, whether of words, or paint, or stone, or mechanic, to which one is native or to which one is trained.

Life is whole, no matter how different the human units of that life are. What they express is later identifiable as characteristic of that life and of the life of no other time. In a very real sense the meaning of this is, that we are not free. No matter to what program for human betterment we wished to dedicate ourselves, to attempt to exercise an influence to that end would be vain and idle, if we ignored the fact of the war now raging. In this crude way there is no escape from being bound to our time. By the same token, any expression, as art, that would attempt the use of the forms of Puvis de Chavannes or of George Watts or of Sandro Botticelli would be regarded as antiquarian and anything but vital—certainly not vital in the sense that the narration would have value as interpreting the contemporary scene—that life which we know and feel and the sense of which is urgent and compelling.

Words, the very use of language, requires understanding in this context. The attempt, formerly, so often made to translate into them, what had been said in another medium, in painting or music or sculpture, received close attention by Samuel Isham [1] some thirty years ago. We should say now that to strike an equivalence is rationally impossible—the very choice of another medium is evidence that the precise information to be conveyed is characteristically possible in that medium and not in another. Words, color, form, sound, each of them affords an opportunity not to be found in the other and accounts for the choice of that precise method of conveyance. This insistence on precision in the choice of medium arises also in that persistent, scientific temper of the Century. I am not saying that in other eras an effort at the exact use of language was not made, but merely that correspondence between what language can convey, and what another form of

[1] *The Limitations of Verbal Criticism of Works of Art*, Portland, Maine, 1928.

expression, was something to which users of language, if not sensitive to the extent that this is possible, are likely, as Isham pointed out, to attempt what is in essence unattainable.

For many persons it has always been a source of great perturbation to find incomprehensible the words so often used by critics and lovers of the pictorial arts. Not to discover their meaning is the more baffling when one harbors the deep conviction that something is occurring which, if translated into language having an appropriate content or accent, would be communicable. It may of course be that in the domain of feeling, of tone, of merely being, there are values without dimensions—that for the mood which these things are, there is required a very special language of conveyance or perhaps no language at all. But in this case, there would be the utmost use in possessing a vocabulary in which such states of feeling can be conveyed—unless there were a method, the existence of which I very much doubt, of communication in which articulateness is quite dispensable and mutual understanding established without the need of identifying the subject of appreciation and of mutual concern.

In this picture of the wholeness of this life, its history, the temper of the times, the use of language, what science is and the part it has played needs to be fairly apprehended. It is perhaps daring to assert that science is no more than the single analytical enterprise of man. Science is analysis and perhaps only one thing more —conception. Conception in this sense is a part merely of apprehension—apprehension of the universe or of as small a section of it as you please. A challenge to being understood on its part, the will to undertake the enterprise of understanding and to carry out the intention by analysis *is* the scientific enterprise. It is entirely idle to try to maintain that nothing else is involved in a successful prosecution of the endeavor—but the rest is mechanics, itself requiring genius but not conceptually relevant.

A little more in detail, science is that activity which dissects nature, which wishes to see, not how nature looks, not what nature is, but essentially how nature works. To find that out is in many situations so difficult that instead of viewing nature or some part of it as a whole, a portion only—like a heart or an eye, or a muscle or a nerve—must serve alone as the object of analysis or study or experiment. Experiment is a special form of inquiry. You do not, for example, know how a structure works. You wonder, is it this way or that; you place that structure in a particular posture or set of postures; you expose it to a variety of environments and you observe the differences in its behavior in each. From that experience or experiences, inferences are drawn which make that working more easily intelligible than would be the case if these procedures, this analysis had not been undertaken.

The word which is to carry the central burden of this discourse is accordingly the word *analysis*. At no time, between the Hellenic age and the rebirth of knowledge, has the process represented by that word received that almost undivided attention that it does now. If fact and the recognition of fact and of factual interrelations are at the core of the scientific attitude, the failure of a philosophy to hold the center of the stage is understandable if that philosophy asserts the nature and structure of things categorically. It would be idle to pretend that Platonism is dead or that its advocates have grown silent, but its success has been challenged during many decades in terms which have insisted on measuring and weighing phenomena and on using statistical methods, to be certain that forecasting the occurrence and recurrence of acts is correct.

That is why in recent years so much of history has taken the course it has. Mommsen has been mentioned. But Toynbee and the meaning of his colossal enterprise should be. Here, applied to history, is an example of the scientific method. The earlier members of the school of exact historicity insisted on establishing the facts of the historical narrative. Documents were wanted and scrupulously sought. They were studied, annotated, arranged, weighed, to yield whatever evidence was needed or was possible in establishing a point of view. Exactness was necessary. What Toynbee has done must be regarded as a step further. In addition to documents, he collected histories of entire societies. Following the example of analytical scientists, these were the crude facts meant to serve the purposes of generalization. Generalization, it is all but unnecessary to mention, is a stage in the mechanics of scientific investigation for which the fact finding and fact collecting stages are preliminary and indispensable. This is the stage in which, having made analyses, the effort is made to arrive at a simple statement, called a law, to cover or designate the whole experience. The search for fact and the arrangement of facts is common to the entire scientific attitude. The laws of nature are the simplest statements, based on fact, that can be found to describe occurrences in the world.

Now to return to the word analysis. But before doing so, perhaps a word on what should not have been expected from the title of this discourse. As everyone knows, in the one hundred and fifty years past, great additions have been made to the sum total of information about many aspects of the work-a-day procedures in painting and sculpture. Of very great importance is the wider knowledge of the chemistry of pigments, of the properties of materials, of gums and resins, of their enduring properties, of luminosity, qualities of surface. These are all matters entering into the business of representation which have their very great importance in craftsmanship. But they are matters of technology. They have not to do with the description of principles and insights and ultimate objectives which are the proper considerations basic to this study.

The road to be traveled in the survey of rational—of analytical —performance in painting encounters milestones labeled impressionism at the beginning, and at the end, expressionism. Along the road other milestones are labeled post-impressionism, cubism, futurism, vorticism, Dadaism, Tatlinism, synchromism. The array of designations is startling and disconcerting as if each name, each milestone represents something new in the realm of possible, new, independently conjectured, efforts in creative imagination.

Out of the past came, in painting, an inheritance in which whatever experiment was made, the assumption was always tacit that the major effort was to convey what the eyes saw in the outside world, after having passed with a minimum of distortion or transformation in the mind of the artist to the finished canvas there to be scrutinized by the eyes of the beholder. That was, more or less, the theory. The emphasis was on the outside world.

Without doubt changes in theory had always been taking place. A simple chronological table is Mr. Baldwin Brown's:

(i) up to and including the Egyptians—the time of the search for Truth of Contour. The Egyptians in their flat silhouettes achieved a perfection of contour which has never been surpassed; (ii) from the Egyptians to the Fifteenth Century—the time of "the struggle for three dimensions," or Truth of Form; (iii) the Fifteenth and Sixteenth Centuries—the culmination of the struggle, when victory was won through a proper appreciation of perspective; (iv) after the Sixteenth Century—the "search for the wider horizon"—Truth of Space. Practically the whole of French painting falls within the last two periods, and it therefore had to take its part in the struggle for Truth of Form and Truth of Space.[2]

These divisions in the time schedule—to the Egyptians; thence to the 15th Century; then the 15th and 16th Centuries; and finally after the 16th, became constantly and increasingly shorter. More change has taken place between 1819 (the birth of Courbet) and roughly 1890, in seventy years than in the whole of the preceding record. The passage is from impressionism to expressionism. If the obvious interest of painters had been presentation, change with astonishing acceleration occurred. And the impetus for this, as I have been trying to say, was conditioned by the temper of the time characterized by nothing so much as attention to nature with the accuracy contributed by science. Everybody, everywhere has been bent on the same enterprise. The temper and the tempo which scientists have set this age are formidable—in thought and industry and in politics—all of a piece. This was not the first epoch though in which rational methods were employed in improving the art of representation—the study of perspective and of the anatomy of the surface of the human body are evidence to the contrary. It is, as many critics believe, owing to the great curiosity and insight of painters—of Leonardo especially—of the Calcar-Vesalius combination, of

[2] *A Short History of French Painting*, Eric G. Underwood, Oxford, 1931, p. 274.

Michelangelo, that greater accuracy in rendering the form of the surface of the body took place.

But now wholly new motives entered the calculation—the new contributions of physics, of chemistry, of photography, of psychology as represented in the great revolution by the assertion that individual men and women had value. These discoveries and assertions changed the face of things in painting and sculpture so that that progression along the road, the road that has been traveled —became all but inevitable.

That word inevitable gives one pause. It is as if it were correct to believe this is the best of all possible worlds—as if, if painters and sculptors reached a decision and took a course, no other one were possible; as if there were no exhibitionists, no charlatans, no· exploiters; as if it were possible, under the dominant and compelling influences of a time, to escape from applying to one's own activity the techniques and motives everyone else was applying, not understanding that these motives and techniques were inapplicable to the methods intrinsically appropriate to one's own activity. Restlessness and adventure, always with us, and especially imminent now, compel change. There is, and was, perhaps no choice but to try. There is after all no risk—except that to the integrity of the intellectual process—and time cures error there. As will appear, under the influence of the *Zeitgeist*, painters and sculptors, imported into their arts, forces, some of which had extraordinary success and will no doubt, in some measure, remain permanent contributions to the craft. But others of these forces, like bombs, were disturbing incidents, destroying rather than making grow. How this may be becomes evident on examining certain aspects of the artistic enterprise.

In an art, at least three elements cannot escape being ingredient. One is, what is that art about; a second is, with what means is that art conveyed; and a third is, what attitude is taken to the two others? It is unnecessary to make a category of the arts. It is unnecessary, furthermore, to estimate the place or the function an art or the arts occupy or serve in the entire scheme of things. Custom, in a rough way, suggests what an art is. And yet that is an escape from precision—for many aspects of human activity, beside the arts proper, exhibit an artistic component. We will leave them aside.

But of those human activities which it is customary to regard as arts, painting and sculpture surely are two. Their subject matter or, to repeat the less differentiated expression, what they are about, concerns something in the outside world—usually, because now what originates in the world of the mind may also be admitted as subject matter, though it makes little difference whether it is "admitted." If an artist chooses to paint what goes on there (in his mind) no one will interfere. If he succeeds in finding an audience—art or no art, his activity will receive comment, his product will find a niche in the records of his time, irrespective of any scholastic view of its appropriateness. The professors have often judged wrong. Of course, what goes on in the mind may be limited to the mind's use of the impressions conveyed to it from the outside world. There may be no other source for impressions. To believe this after Berkeley is still proper doctrine. Indeed there may exist between the two worlds, inner and outer, the most intimate sort of organic relation. What the art, originating in the mind, is about, is, in short, about the same world, the inner and the outer, differing only by the degree to which an artist impresses his person on the new material of the outside, the "real" world. The two worlds are in essence, therefore, one.

For the sake of simplicity, it will be to painting that these remarks apply.

Now the second element. In painting obviously there is a vast choice of means available for conveying an artist's intention; size of the presentation, its precise subject, the method and intention of the drawing of that subject, the color and light with which it is endowed.

And third, the attitude an artist takes to the first two—the subject matter and the choice of the technique of presentation. Clearly there can be no presentation in which one of the two elements can be omitted. But there is a choice on what to do or how to think and feel. And clearly that choice consists in the emphasis which is placed on subject or technique—whether what matters more is subject or method. It is aside the point to insist that when, as literary critics point out in the case of Sophocles or Shakespeare, great success is attained, it is a happy blend of the two. The difficulty is, the subject varies and, as will become apparent, so does the technique—with time. In fact, the degree to which subject matter has been depressed to a level of second interest has been, especially in recent painting, frequently commented upon. It is a fact though that the 19th Century saw a vast extension of interest in the presentation of certain phases of outdoors—interest in painting *en plein air*. But whether this performance was primary or depended on the opportunity for the study of light and color is an important consideration. It is at this point that what part science occupied in the evolution of painting, enters.

When Courbet flourished, photography began to come into vogue. Young had already been speculating on light and its perception by the eye. And in the middle of the century, Helmholtz published his *Handbook of Physiological Optics*. Out of these elements developed on the scientific side the motives which have dominated painting ever since. But science in the form of sociology made a further contribution. In analyzing the lives of ordinary men and women it succeeded in making evident where, in our scheme of things, the processes of industry, industry itself being the foster child of applied science, left much to be desired in providing for their life, liberty and their pursuit of happiness. In European and American painting both, in Millet, Daumier, Grant Wood, Rivera, the results of historical and social analysis are plentifully evident.

But of these two components, physics or physiology and sociology, painters turned their attention first to the former. They did in fact to a great extent neglect the latter. They deserted an interest in philanthropy, the struggles of men in society and their contest with nature and devoted themselves to what could be seen. Courbet contributed powerfully to this movement in such statements as these:

Painting is an art of sight and should concern itself with things seen; it should, therefore, abandon both the historical scenes of the Classical school and poetic subjects from Goethe and Shakespeare favoured by the Romantic school. . . .

Painting is a wholly physical language, and an invisible or abstract thing is not within its province. Our grandiose painting is a contradiction of our social conditions, our church painting of the spirit of the age. It is an absurdity for painters to trot out subjects in which they have no real interest and which are appropriate to a time and place remote from our own. It is far better to paint railway stations . . . engine houses, mines and factories. These are the saints and miracles of the Nineteenth Century.[3]

The movement which embraced these admonitions became known as "impressionism." It will be desirable later to understand such designating terms, which have a function not in themselves but of indicating the milestones already referred to on a road along which there was continuous evolution; once attention was almost exclusively linked to the technique of vision.

The break with the naturalism of the past, with facts themselves, was sharp. Narrative, information, organization and structure in painting became distinctly secondary. Rendering light and color became primary interests. And even light and color and such interest as there was in the subject was broken down still further in the interest of scientific simplicity. Out of doors, in its travel, the light of the sun and the shadows which are cast, are in process of continuous change. To document the variety of effect resulting from changes in illumination according to time of day or to season, Monet painted a long series of haystacks. This point was in fact driven so far as to limit the period of painting to a space of time during which the quality or the effect of the light remained uniform. Obviously under such an influence it was but a short distance to the conclusion that the first or any other single subsequent impression of an object could or should be the subject of representation. The instantaneous impression was the observation of value. Representation which involved continuity or enduring existence was impossible.

There was a literary counterpart to this view illustrated by the slice of life method adopted by Zola and his followers. Whatever

[3] *A Short History of French Painting*, Eric G. Underwood, Oxford, 1931, p. 243.

one saw, became important—beauty or ugliness, it mattered not which. Life consisted of instantaneous pictures. It was about these that it was desirable to know.

The interest in color and in vision went on its way. Everyone knows that color outdoors and color indoors differs vastly. But the difference which was now emphasized was new. Color outdoors was bright. The problem was, how was this appearance to be reproduced. The current scientific investigations led the way. White light, the light of the sun was now known to be broken into certain colors which were observed when white light passed through a prism—the arrangement of colors forming a band ranging from infrared—the colors made of the longest wave lengths—to ultraviolet, those that are made of the shortest wave lengths. When these are recombined they make white light. It was a gratifying, confirming observation that this breakdown of white light into prismatic colors was observable also in outdoor nature, in the rainbow. It was a stimulating discovery. The way in which proof was offered was ingenious. On a disc of paper divided into shapes like the triangular pieces into which we cut pies, appropriate colors were applied. When the paper so prepared was rotated fast enough, the colors blended and the result was again white light—or almost white. The distinction between primary and secondary colors now needed to be recognized. Primary colors were such as appeared in the spectrum and which, when combined, any two of them made other colors. The colors of the spectrum, between red and violet were, according to Newton, orange, yellow, green, blue and indigo. Rotating all the spectral colors gives the appearance of white light. But another arrangement is possible. Two selected colors when painted on halves of a piece of circular paper will when rotated do it. Red and green are such colors, or yellow and blue. Such pairs are known as complementary colors. There are many others. What was also noticed was that an effect of greater luminosity was created or at least greater brillance in effect, when two such complementary colors were placed side by side. When this discovery was made and the effect properly understood, the way was prepared for the course painting was to take for a couple of generations. To the exclusion of almost every other interest, attention was now riveted on the problems of light, at least to the extent that light entered into the calculation of painters. Subject matter—reform of social abuses, history, literary matters, all fell into a place of second consideration. Locomotives, bathers, machinery, anything in nature or in the city streets became the subject of curiosity—so that it offered opportunities to test out theories of light and the uses to which the application of such theories could be put. And not only light itself, but the medium through which light passed—the atmosphere. The atmosphere received in fact most exact scrutiny; the renderings of it, introduced into pictorial art, turned out to be effects not previously secured, brilliant, befogged, sunlit, colorful, mysterious.

This interest in color affected powerfully the methods commonly used to indicate form. The simplest and the most usual way to bound a form had been the use of line. But now it turned out to be possible to dispense with lines and to replace them with color—color of varying intensity and shade. Comparable techniques had already been introduced by engravers. And in sculpture in a most interesting manner outlines were indicated in bas reliefs. That technique had been exquisitely utilized in the sculptured friezes and panels and other decorations on the walls of the temples in and about Angkor Wat. The use of the new plan of delimitation aided powerfully in stimulating the tactile sense, giving weight to the human body and to other ponderable masses.

These were the first fruits derived from the new interest in light. But an idea like this, once having been born, marches on, evolves as it were out of its own inner existence. Knowledge of the effects to be derived from complementary colors led to testing how in other connections these color impressions could be utilized. A way was soon found in which color was applied to canvas in patches, as a mosaic or as if it were deposited as would be a sprinkling of confetti. And the reason for resort to this plan was the desire to capture that brilliance which was lost when pigments, pigments being after all something different from pure colors, were mixed. Mixing pigments on a palette yielded new colors, but in the process brightness was lost. Now if, instead of mixing them beforehand and then applying them they were laid on side by side, the effect aimed at was attained. But for this effect the spectator must remove himself to an appropriate distance from the canvas. His eyes then make a synthesis of complementary colors into a heightened effect, the result of a combining of the elementary colors in the retina of the eye. What would otherwise have been dull, now became brilliant. This method of laying on complementary colors to gain this effect went by a variety of names, "divisionism," "pointillism," and the "confetti method." Putting down points of color makes possible the heightening of effect wherever it is desired, by inserting a spot of color, yellow or green, where this is needed. This general practice came to be known as "neo-impressionism."

In addition to the gift of color, science made another contribution. It made possible a further departure in the thinking of painters. Disinterest in anecdote and narrative and the absorbing interest in analyzing color led the way to a contraction of curiosity about the outside world. Description was limited as I have suggested to what could be observed in a moment of time. Nature, and what the eye could see, was restricted to the kind of experience that could be gained as it were in a flash. What was inadvertently left out of the totality of experience was the outlook upon the world that could be contributed by the play of the imagination and the operation of the mind of man.

Daumier, Cézanne, Renoir were the new men. Concern for light, concern for form, for meaning, for human insight, received new emphasis. It was a rich time. The insistent development of photography pointed to the impoverishment painting had suffered. Impressionism, like photography, captured only a moment of the scene. Technically painting was not so accurate but from the viewpoint of gaiety it added color. But to add color was not enough. Other tensions, the critical tensions, demanded their own satisfaction and releases. Interest in the fate of men and what was wrong with the human scheme began again to inform the canvasses of men who had now time to recapture an interest in social affairs. Mere representation turned out to be seriously wanting in important interests. But even on the side of representation there

were new things to do. To that concern Cézanne returned, trying
to find novel ways of picturing solid designs—trying to convey
the impression of weight, depth and solidity. It was the solidity
and the implications of solidity with its stress on geometrical arrangement that made of this aspect of Cézanne's adventure a
motive to which later the cubists turned.

Those influences which originated in a belief in the efficacy of
the analytical procedure, the scientific method, were an important
part of the current climate of opinion. They contributed a background for the cubist formulation. Beauty had been playing, conceptually, a relatively small part in the theory and practice of
impressionism. It came in now for renewed attention. Straight lines
were dogmatically asserted to form the essence of beauty. Straight
lines suggested the use of simple form, and made of crystals which
are so often bounded by straight lines, the cornerstone of a new
way of looking. Unlike realists, for whom nature was beauty un-
adorned but also unanalyzed; and unlike impressionists for whom
nature from the viewpoint of light at a single instant was something given, though analyzed, to cubists whatever else was accepted
and retained, such as the inheritance from predecessors of light
and color, nature was the better understood in its dynamic relations if solid bodies, including the bodies of men and animals, were
analyzed and were dissected to reveal the multitude of planes that
formed their boundaries. At first cubism went through a "still
life" phase. The anatomy and geometry of bodies was a source
of never-ending wonder; a new opportunity to gain an insight
into the structure of limiting surfaces. Distortion, and the degree
of it, was of little concern. The exciting experience was the experiment of recognizing how a single point of view could be resolved in components. But to the static, there succeeded soon a
dynamic phase—bodies in motion and the impression made on
the mind's eye by planes in motion. Here was a new world,
doubly removed from common sense reality—planes and planes
in motion.

After impressionism and neo-impressionism—post-impressionism.
As has so often been the case, after the new theory of seeing had

been acquired, to do something with the new toy could not be resisted. And so the mere reproduction of nature, with no matter how new a technique, gave way to an effort to find new things to say. Ideas began again to flow. Artists began again to play with observations of the external world. It was regarded as legitimate to impress one's personal view and even one's bias upon what one saw. A painting could become something beside mere reproduction. To express a personal view was a right and a privilege. The movement that sanctified this tendency is known as Expressionism.

It adds nothing to the general point of view which this essay adopts to describe the later developments which were initiated by the movement of impressionism—abstractionism, futurism, vorticism, Dadaism, Tatlinism, synchromism. They went on to develop motives that deal with expression, with motion, with abstraction. An interest in the analysis of vision and of motion continued. But of more dominating importance was an arbitrary insistence upon the ways of personal seeing and of feeling on the part of individual artists. Vorticism was an effort to find the essence of an object, its form during a heightened emotional experience; and synchromism an attempt to fasten to form an appropriate color, the color representing in an object its own particular property or nature. Color came to possess something beyond naturalistic value. Color is the end object to which impressionism and post-impressionism point. Nothing of importance is left or matters save color. Color becomes form, rhythm—becomes everything.

To all of this Dadaism added a literary phase. I find quoted for example this statement by M. André Gide: "What! While our fields, our villages, our cathedrals have suffered so much, our language is to remain untouched! It is important that the mind should not lag behind matter; it has a right, it too, to some ruins. Dada will see to it."

The passage from naturalism to impressionism which has been traced in painting is observable also in sculpture. That progress can be satisfactorily studied in Rodin in the transition from the

Age of Bronze to his John the Baptist. Like the impressionists he too froze into permanent form the experience or the impression of a moment. The same purposes were influential in sculpture as in painting. Impressionism gave place to cubism and expressionism. Travel and exploration, especially African, made way for the introduction of a new freedom so that to attain sculptural effects of mass, essentially sculptural ideas and feeling, prettiness and exact representation were relegated to positions at least of second importance. Distortion, when it gave point to feeling, was employed, and solid mass—these are the qualities which distinguished this sculpture. I avoid the use of words such as rhythm, not uncommonly employed, because a definition of what their precise meaning is, is far from obvious.

From the point of view of scientific consideration sculpture exhibits little that is basically different from painting. Its one clear reflection is in the study of surfaces and here the influence of cubism is apparent. Sculpture does in fact lend itself conspicuously to an experiment in planes.

After expressionism the onward march came to its fulfillment in the pieces of Brancusi. His effort consisted in the search for the essence of an object. This art is termed abstract because all accidental things are removed. And it was in fact, so. What remains suggests an idea, an abstraction. It can be graceful, it can be moving. But very soon a limit seems to be reached. Sculpture may not be the medium for this adventure.

I have come to the end of this necessarily brief account of the influence of science on modern painting and sculpture. It is apparent that this influence has been limited, conspicuously, as perhaps one should expect, to problems of seeing, problems of vision. Since what we see is color, motion, and the qualities of form, it would naturally and necessarily be these that received primary attention. When emotion was expressed by such vehicles as were being used, or when, at least, that form of expression of emotion or perception was undertaken, the result came near to necessitating a written guide of interpretation. The effort to force further and further stuff of the mind, originating as did this material, on artistic techniques initially unequivocal, conceptually—that effort ended in frayed thinking and in frayed nerves.

I have not intended to omit mention of other particulars you may expect to find included here. This is not a catalogue and has no claim to systematic completeness. Without enlarging on each of these matters, I should perhaps refer to those other subjects to which natural science has contributed. At the beginning, when I tried to explain the vast interrelatedness of things, my intention was to emphasize the point that, since the whole of current life is dominated by a positivist, a factual viewpoint, it may not always be possible to identify the underlying scientific objective. Economics and sociology are beginning more and more to be closely identified with scientific methods. Awareness of many less savory sides of American life can readily and insistently have come to public attention by other means; but certain it is that the new methods, in this case the statistical language employed in science, are being used by government and scholars. Certain it is also that much contemporary painting tells the seamy story. This is the contribution of social science to art. The Freudian tradition also without doubt has affected painters. Patterns in dreams, their arrangements and colors have been recollected and reproduced. Such influences have in fact found expression in canvasses in subtle ways, not always known even to the creators themselves.

Zoology and botany and the physical sciences in general have exerted their direct or even their indirect influence. But in these cases where animals are studied, the emphasis is placed on motion rather than on natural history.

Taking it all in all—in special examples and in general—the sum total of the range of subject matter on which scientific influence has been exerted has not been wide, although it has, nevertheless, permeated the major part of modern art. Its use is clear, its future so far ill defined.

It is not unusual for writers or speakers in the absence of professional knowledge or even of amateur status to disclaim all appearance of speaking with authority. I fear I must adopt this formula of inadequacy and remind you that my own path has lain far removed from those fields through which we have been wandering together. I pray that my disclaimer be taken seriously. Contrary to general custom I place it at the end of this discourse. I choose this place so that I may leave my confession of ignorance as the last of the impressions you are to receive. The plan is, in this way, to emphasize my sincerity. I have enjoyed searching my mind and have enjoyed communicating my layman's conception of this important subject.

John Wyckoff: 1881-1937

I HAVE come to pay tribute to the memory of a remarkable man. I knew John Wyckoff in many of the relations common among men in our profession—as a man, as a friend, as a scholar. I called him Jack, as did all his friends—perhaps especially his older friends. That that was natural, bears eloquent testimony to the human and humane qualities with which the diverse aspects of our lives became invested. To John Wyckoff to be human was to err. That conviction provided the latitude which, added to the inelastic rectitude of his own nature, made communication with him on the part of lesser men—not so much possible, but a benediction. I am certain that many men, to obtain his approbation, lived lives on levels they would not otherwise have attained. His sympathy with general human failing saved him from a sense of superiority and the rest of us from a sense of condescension. If I say that to me he seemed great in character, I say no more than I mean. But if I fail to suggest the delightfulness of his companionability, the impression I am conveying falls short of reality.

Wyckoff was born in the Madras presidency (India) and came of a missionary family. For those of us to whom nurture, like Matthew Arnold's conduct, is two-thirds of life, it is natural to derive the elevation of his moral nature from the influences of his earlier environment. A sense of responsibility, a feeling of obligation to leave his own world better than he found it, was a passion he did not so much as express, though he did that too, as made evident to the observers of his career, in the course along which he steered his life. Innumerable acts along that course serve the function of buoys that indicate the channel along which he sailed his craft. A sense of responsibility—a feeling of obligation. These qualities are not enough, however, with which to characterize his deep-lying motives. Wyckoff was a profoundly purposeful man.

He loved men and beyond that, he loved justice among men. Good intentions, he required. Once he was convinced they had that, equality of opportunity, irrespective of race, creed, or color, were not merely conventional, obfuscating terms. Fair dealing was for him an obsessing reality. If he had no presentiments beyond the immediate implications of these views, it was because he did not choose to explore them, believing as I know he did, that to attempt to foresee, in the too distant future, all the consequences of his acts, was to subordinate the impulse of generosity to the chilling effect of design. He had a shrewd sense that in certain regions of behavior "diplomacy is too much for man." To act as these beliefs required him to act was to exhibit how a nobleman fulfilled the function of a democrat. A world fashioned after his pattern would be a tolerable place in which to live.

He carried his general intentions in respect to living, into professional existence. He meant to leave that better than he found it—in practice; in education, which is preparation for practice; in his care of the public health, which is practice for the common man; and in research, which is preparation, ultimately, for practice.

I am certain the possession of power was not a dominant motive with him. The possession of power was mere incident to his purpose. I have never heard that he exercised it except with the utmost restraint. I have never heard that men regarded his use of it in any sense other than benevolent. As proof, I can cite the unusual size of his following among his younger colleagues. To them, to be one of Wyckoff's men meant, not the limitation, but the fruitful development, of their powers. Wyckoff knew how to share power and how to delegate it—not with the view to sparing himself, but so as to acquaint as many men as possible with the technique of its exercise. The evidence for the complete success of his plan and the proof that he knew how to put it into operation is that this School, over which he presided so brief a time, received from him an impress so directive and so powerful as to render all but unnecessary more, for the moment, than a steering hand. I say for the moment, for in the troubled seas of our world, the course of any ship cannot be left to chance, but will require frequently to be recalculated. But this can confidently be said—

the conception to which he made it conform, because it was informed with breadth and was founded on profound general principles, has vitality, vivacity and, I hope and believe, durability.

He touched the life of medicine on many sides. To that group
of diseases to which he devoted his thinking especially, he imparted new energy. He came to the study of cardio-vascular diseases at a time when, what seemed to be their increase, was engaging, in this city, the apprehensive attention of physicians. It is
relatively simple to trace his share in events which, though they
evolved in an orderly fashion, can be seen now to have constituted
a genuine revolution in conceptions entertained of this group of
diseases. The importance which this subject presents may be gauged
by the reflection that cardiac diseases are by far the greatest problem presented to students of the public health in our country.
Wyckoff's interest in them began in 1909 in Bellevue Hospital,
on rounds with Dr. Hermann Biggs. Dr. Biggs had been speaking
of the problems connected with heart disease and especially of
those of rheumatic fever for which convalescent homes, vocational
guidance and beds for the permanently disabled were wanted. "Dr.
Bigg's last words that day," Wyckoff writes, "I remember well.
'The time is not ripe yet to make rheumatic fever a reportable disease, but the time will come when it will be made reportable.' "

Almost thirty years have passed but that time has not come even
yet. If it does, and I hope it may soon, not the least contribution
to that consummation will have been Wyckoff's. The method he
pursued was intricate and time-consuming, but it has been effective and has made his enduring reputation. His method was the
method developed in the cardiac clinic. His method, in fact, *was*
the cardiac clinic. It is to the lasting glory of the Bellevue Hospital
and of this School, that this achievement took place here. Here
was something new under the sun. There is no general realization even now how far-reaching are the ideas that were then conceived nor how fundamental to future developments, already in
sight. Wyckoff built on a foundation which already had been laid
—a firm foundation, for it was built in response to a positive social
need. Miss Wadley has just written to me (February 9, 1938)

what she remembers of the very beginning. It was she, so far as
I can learn, to whom the idea came.

"It is quite true," she tells me, "that the initial move in establishing
this clinic belongs to Bellevue Social Service. Scores of cardiacs discharged from the wards were referred to Social Service for convalescent
care and for assistance in finding suitable employment. This we could
do but continued medical oversight was imperative if they were to
carry on. For most of them this oversight was obtainable only in the
day clinics and day clinics and jobs were incompatible. The situation
was most distressing to patients, physicians and to the hospital. We
social workers knew that the solution for a large proportion of cases
could be found in a special evening clinic, but there was prejudice
against evening clinics. Dr. Hubert Guile was deeply interested in
these cases and he agreed to give his time to directing an evening clinic if
the hospital authorities would consent to the innovation. They did consent to it as an *experiment*.[1] This was in 1911, and there has practically
been no Friday evening at Bellevue since then without a Cardiac Clinic
Session. We chose Friday for the clinic as that would give the patient
a two-day rest, if needed, with the loss of only half a working day
and he could be back on the job Monday morning before a new
worker could replace him. Our Social Service Committee was greatly
interested and contributed the salary of a full-time special worker.
After devoting his time for several years to this clinic, Dr. Guile felt
he must retire. He had interested many young physicians in the opportunity the clinic afforded for an intensive study of heart disease. Dr.
John Wyckoff had been one of the most interested assistants and he
was persuaded to take Dr. Guile's place. He threw himself into the
further development of the work with great zeal and was influential
in the establishment of many similar evening clinics elsewhere." [2]

[1] "A Survey of the Bellevue Experiment in Preventive Work for 'Cardiacs,'" by Katharine Tyng, in *Bellevue
and Allied Hospitals Social Service Reports*, 1910-1914, is available at the
New York Academy of Medicine.
[2] On October 7, 1942, Mary E.
Wadley died in Albany, N. Y., in the
fullness of her 90 years. Her passing
off the scene ought not to fail of being
recorded. In the history of the development of interest in cardiac diseases

Miss Wadley played an important even
if not a conspicuous part. She was the
first one to recognize the fact that
cardiac patients were receiving less care
than they deserve or than it was possible to give to them. Miss Wadley was
head of the Social Service Department
of the Bellevue Hospital in New York
City. What she did was to create for
the Bellevue Hospital Social Service a
cardiac clinic for working adults. She
saw the need and stimulated Dr. Hubert

There is good evidence that with this account of the role played by the Social Service in this movement, Wyckoff would wholeheartedly have agreed. He insisted upon designating this clinic "Bellevue Hospital Social Service Cardiac Clinic for Working Adults," for this was the title of the clinic when it was turned over to him in 1919 by Dr. Guile. Miss Lingg recalls that Wyckoff was determined to maintain this as its correct title. In his plan of organization the Social Service was the center from which all action moved and to which all action returned. In 1925, when he described the organization of cardiac clinics to the Medical Society of the State of New York,[3] the position of the Social Service at the center of things was conspicuously indicated. And he repeated these statements in 1929.

"The first cardiac clinic in the United States as a matter of fact was organized at Bellevue Hospital in 1911 by Dr. H. V. Guile at the request of Miss Wadley, the head of the Social Service Department, who felt the pressing need for the medical supervision of the ambulatory cardiac. In 1919 I took over this clinic, having during the preceding eight years worked in it at various times." [4]

V. Guile to undertake the creation of the Friday evening clinic. The movement which she brought into being can most fittingly be described in her own words in a letter written by her on February 9, 1938. (See p. 64.) One of the pities in recording the lives of persons and the history of movements is frequently the paucity of information that is available. But in this instance by good chance the beginning is known of an important matter. The care of patients suffering from cardiac diseases moved, through Miss Wadley's insight and interest, into a new era. If there were cardiac clinics at all or cardiac clinics having a purpose such as this one before the one at Bellevue Hospital, it is unknown to me. And so both to record the beginning of a valuable movement as well as to commemorate the name of Mary E. Wadley, a distinguished worker in this vineyard of the Lord, it is gratifying to record this piece of history. ("The First Cardiac Clinic," *Jour. Amer. Med. Assn.*, 1943, *121*, p. 70.)

[3] "The first clinic in this country for ambulatory cardiacs was established in 1911, by Dr. Hubert V. Guile, in Bellevue Hospital. It was begun because the Social Service Department of the hospital felt that the number of returns of cardiac patients to the wards could be diminished if the patients could, upon discharge, be cared for in a clinic less crowded than the General Medical Clinic, and manned by physicians who would have time to become interested in the special problems of the heart patient." *N. Y. State J. Med.*, 1925, *25*, 995-1001 (p. 996).

[4] "A Consideration of Causes of Heart Disease from the Standpoint of a Social Worker," *Hosp. Social Service*, 1929, *19*, 513-24 (p. 514).

I begin this description of Wyckoff's scientific career at this point designedly, because, it seems certain, whatever followed had its origin here. After the first impetus given him by Dr. Biggs, emphasized during a visit to Bad Nauheim in the summer of 1909 (Bellevue Violet) or 1910, he joined Dr. Guile (1914-1915) in the conduct of the Social Service Cardiac Clinic, until he accepted a commission in the U. S. Army in 1918 (February). On his return in 1919 he rejoined Dr. Guile who in this same year turned over the clinic to him.

Meanwhile others in New York, including Dr. Guile, moved by the plight of cardiac patients, started an organization for their care. This organization, the Association for the Prevention and Relief of Heart Disease, began its movement in 1915 but was obliged to suspend activities during the period of the War (1917-1919). In 1920 (January 20) Wyckoff was elected to membership.

In 1917 (February) the heart association called into being the Association of Cardiac Clinics. Six years later, in 1923 (April 27), the Association of Cardiac Clinics became an integral part of the Association for the Prevention and Relief of Heart Disease and was called the Committee on Cardiac Clinics. Dr. William P. St. Lawrence was Chairman, but later in the same year (November 26, 1923) Wyckoff succeeded him. The Association for the Prevention and Relief of Heart Disease (its name meanwhile changed to the New York Heart Committee) joined the New York Tuberculosis and Health Association in the early months of 1926.[5]

When precisely the methods of examination and of diagnosis in use in the Bellevue Cardiac Clinic were adopted I have been unable to learn. But I have a manila envelope, dated 1919, on which is printed the form of diagnosis then employed. It reflected the view, then altogether novel, that a cardiac diagnosis to be

[5] For a record of Wyckoff's relations with the various organizations concerned with cardiac patients see *Bulle-* *tin of the Institute of the History of Medicine*, 1938, vi, p. 840.

reasonably complete, required a three-fold description. Wyckoff adopted three headings:

A. Anatomical
B. Functional and
C. Etiology

The folders within the envelope are likewise printed and arranged in such a way that relevant data could be filled in, in the blank spaces.

Under what circumstances, simple, single diagnoses of cardiac diseases were found to be inadequate is not wholly clear. Obviously the success that attended the discovery of the etiological relation of microorganisms to infectious diseases was important. That conception underlay Cabot's contention (1914) as well as that entertained by the authors of the circulatory section in Nelson's Loose Leaf Medicine (1920). It was also apparent that between pathological anatomical diagnoses and clinical phenomena there was very disturbing incongruence. And finally, increasing knowledge of cardiac mechanisms made apparent that, irrespective of cause or structure, phenomena appeared which could not be subsumed under either of them. The time had obviously come for making classifications which, even if temporary, facilitated description. This being the state of affairs, it is not remarkable that it occurred to several persons synchronously to find a way out of this dilemma. The situation seems to have been similar to that in which simultaneous discoveries have become familiar. Already in 1919, Wyckoff was dividing cardiac diagnosis into anatomical, functional, and etiological phases, as is shown in his manila envelopes. Under etiology he distinguished 1. Syphilis, 2. Rheumatic Fever and 5. Senility (and also 3. Other acute infections, 4. Alcohol, and 6. Other). In the following years, during 1920 and 1921, in the studies that were being made in preparing the clinical charts recommended by the Association for the Prevention and Relief of Heart Disease, the plan of entering separate diagnoses was incorporated. The earliest specimens written out in pencil still survive and demonstrate the evolution of a two-fold into a three-fold form. Space was assigned in them for etiological, anatomical, and functional diagnoses. These charts were reproduced in the Journal of the American Medical Association in May, 1922.[6]

The Committee on Cardiac Clinics of the New York Association for the Prevention and Relief of Heart Disease continued to be active in elaborating its studies of the proper management of such clinics. In 1923, William St. Lawrence, Chairman of the Committee, Wyckoff being a member, published "Requirements for an ideal cardiac clinic and a system of nomenclature."[7] The diagnosis recommended was now four-fold, comprising etiology, structure, pathological physiology, and functional capacity. Two years after Wyckoff introduced his new conception, White and Myers[8] published (29th October 1921) a scheme in which the main divisions were etiology, structural change and functional condition. In general this arrangement resembled Wyckoff's original form but differed from it in being somewhat fuller. They adopted in addition the plan of the New York Association of Cardiac Clinics of functional grouping.[9]

In this clinic Wyckoff found ways of utilizing the various resources that were available—physicians, nurses, social services, medical services and other medical departments. It was a complete organization for the care of the cardiac sick, inside and outside of hospital. What was wanting and necessary, was a method for analyzing the multitude of data that were obtained. This want was made good by the statistical clerks of the Research Committee

[6] "Clinical Charts Recommended by the Association for the Prevention and Relief of Heart Disease." Alfred E. Cohn. *Jour. Amer. Med. Assn.*, 1922, *78*, 1559-62.

[7] *Boston Med. and Surg. Jour.*, 1923, *189*, 762-68.

[8] P. D. White and M. M. Myers. "The Classification of Cardiac Diagnosis," *Jour. Amer. Med. Assn.*, 1921, *77*, 1414-15.

[9] In a footnote to Cohn's paper this statement was made: "The method of diagnosis advised by the A. P. R. H., has already been published in a paper by White, P. D., and Myers, M. M. . . ." This means, if I remember correctly, that White and Myers published their paper, the form having already been in use in the Association for the Prevention and Relief of Heart Disease. In a letter to Wyckoff, White writes: ". . . I feel quite sure from a visit to your clinic about that year at Bellevue you were also working on this same idea of the classification of cardiac diagnoses, but I can't find in the literature any publication of yours until the one with Lingg in the *American Heart Journal* in 1926." (November 6, 1936.)

of the Association for the Prevention and Relief of Heart Disease, and the use of the statistical charts. This service had recently, beginning in 1920, been in process of formation and was gladly put at the disposal of his clinic, early in 1923. Miss Mebane, the sole statistical clerk at that time reported [10] that she had made a "chart to show the effect of rheumatic fever, chorea, and tonsillitis upon longevity." As is well known, the conception which underlay the statistical service had a two-fold origin—first, the need that was felt of increasing immediately, the very meager information available in the classification (or etiology) of the cardiac diseases; and second, the method, derived from the practice of the U. S. Army Medical Corps, of collecting for later analysis, duplicates of soldiers' field cards. This is not the time to describe the evolution, in 1920, in the research section of Dr. R. H. Halsey's Committee on Prevention, in the Association for the Prevention and Relief of Heart Disease, of the form of the Army field card into the now familiar cardiac chart. Of the charts there is a long history which I will not narrate now. It required little persuasion for Wyckoff to appreciate the value of the method. In his first paper [11] published with Miss Lingg, he commended it in these words:

". . . Owing to the successful results in the use of the charts in a clinical system suitably organized, we are encouraged in the belief that the future success of collecting data on the subject of organic heart disease is assured. After a somewhat tedious transition period from a simpler form of record, previously employed in the clinic, to the new form, it was found that the use of the charts increases rather than decreases the efficiency of the clinic. In fact, after two years' experience, it is our opinion that the provisions made in the chart for recording facts exactly, in the form of a code rather than in the form of a narrative and diagrammatic description, has made it possible (1) to spend more time on the patient and less on the record, while at the same time the important points revealed by the examination have been completely recorded; (2) to see more patients at each session than

[10] July and August (1923?).
[11] "Statistical Studies Bearing on Problems in the Classification of Heart Diseases. II. Etiology in Organic Heart Disease." J. Wyckoff and C. Lingg. *Am. Heart J.*, 1926, I, 446-70.

would otherwise have been possible, and (3) to collate the experience obtained for study and analysis with a minimum expenditure of time and effort."

Later, in 1925, he advocated for still further and wider use, a plan which he himself had found serviceable:

"Since heart disease," he wrote, "is chronic and observations are made frequently over a considerable period of years, and as memory is short, it is essential that all observations should be written down upon a record. They should be noted as briefly as is consistent with accuracy, and the system of notation should be as uniform as possible: First, as to the location of information on the chart, so that one knows where to turn to find such information, and second, as to nomenclature, so that as far as possible, similar observations and procedures will always be described in the same way. Furthermore, from the standpoint of the cardiac problem as a whole all cardiac clinics should use the same record form, the same nomenclature and criteria for diagnosis; otherwise it will be impossible to gather together the data from all clinics for statistical study. The necessity for statistical study cannot be overstressed. Many fundamental questions concerning heart disease can be answered by no other means. Modern medical principles of treating the patient as a whole require that all the records of each out-patient be filed together. A central record system needs good administrative management in order to be effective, but it is far superior to the old plan in which each special clinic had its independent record filed by itself. If such a record system is used, all cardiac diagnoses must be indexed and cross-indexed if they are to be of real use as a source of information." [12]

The relation between the clinic and the Heart Association became so close and interdependent that when, during the great depression, the funds of the Research Committee became depleted, Wyckoff offered financial support to assure a continuation of the service. This support ($300) was gladly accepted as a token of the value of the service rendered by the Research Committee.

The value which he himself attached to the cardiac clinic is

[12] "The Organization of the Cardiac Clinic," *N. Y. State Jour. Med.*, 1925, 25, 995-1001 (p. 999).

made evident by the four publications which he devoted to it.[13] The problems which he encountered in the management of ambulatory patients led him to further reflection on how this task could be properly performed. He saw that their interests would be better served if they were entrusted to the care of a *single* physician who would be responsible for giving advice and prescribing treatment, not only in the clinic but in the hospital ward itself. He was led to advocate, therefore, single control of the entire machinery which ministered to the care of each patient. How he expanded his clinic to serve the actual requirements of patients so that their therapeutic management would be certain to be appropriate to the exact form of their cardiac disease, need not be recapitulated here. It was an extraordinary exhibition in mastery of that form of organization, and very justly made the Bellevue Hospital Cardiac Clinic known far beyond the confines of this land. I should not fail to mention in this connection the care and the interest he took in imparting his own solicitude to his associates. The addresses he made to Nurses and to Social Service Workers in 1924, and 1929, and in 1931, bear witness to his sense of dependence upon them and his confidence that this reliance was not misplaced. The accomplishments of the clinic were manifold—first, in the successful treatment of the sick; second, in the education of students, young and old (in recent years my own associates, Steele, Lewis, and Holman have been devoted learners and helpers); and third, in the advancement of knowledge. In a typewritten report of 1932, I find his statement that about 30 papers had emanated from this clinic. I am given to understand there are now about 67.

In all this Wyckoff took a dominant part. He saw that to make progress, knowledge and still more knowledge was necessary. It began to be recognized that heart disease was not a unit, that

[13] "Organization of the Cardiac Clinic." J. Wyckoff and W. W. O'Conner. *Hosp. Social Service*, 1922, v. 309-16. "Requirements for an Ideal Cardiac Clinic and a System of Nomenclature." W. St. Lawrence, E. P. Maynard, H. E. B. Pardee, M. A. Rothschild, J. Wyckoff. *Bost. Med. Surg. Jour.*, 1923, *189*, 762-68. "The Organization of the Cardiac Clinic." J. Wyckoff. *N. Y. State Jour. Med.*, 1925, 25, 995-1001. "How the Cardiac Clinic Helps the Patient." J. Wyckoff. *Mod. Hospital*, 1926, xxvii, 68-70.

instead there were many, or at all events, several diseases of the heart. Well do I remember how, in committee, it was necessary to do battle for the notion that it was no more fitting to refer to heart disease, than it was correct to designate diseases of the lungs as lung disease. If that were so, it became essential to discover which were the significant cardiac diseases. Wyckoff fell in at once with the idea that the method of trial and error alone, the method designated empiricism, was competent to yield the information that was desired. Patients in large numbers required to be examined and catalogued to discover the variety of groups into which they fell and, in order to discover the relative, social importance of the various classes, the numbers exhibiting each variety. Meanwhile, to make the necessary distinctions, language, terms adequate to the purpose, was developed, and definitions universally understood by physicians engaged in these studies. Something of the history of this phase of the movement has already been described.

In this clinic it was demonstrated that research of first-rate quality, having as its object the description of the natural history of various cardiac diseases, could be undertaken and completed with success. Wyckoff himself with Miss Claire Lingg published the first investigation, from which I have already quoted, under the joint happy auspices of the clinic and the New York Heart Association. Theirs was the first full-dress publication dealing with such matters in this country. Naturally, there were predecessors. There always are. But these did no more than vaguely to indicate a way. In their report, the numerical relations of youthful and senescent cardiac diseases was pointed out and the demonstration clearly made to what extent it was rheumatic fever that accounted for disability in the young and something else—arteriosclerosis perhaps—which accounted for it in the old. What was learned was that roughly between three- and four-tenths of the cases were rheumatic, four-tenths areteriosclerotic, one-tenth syphilitic and all other varieties, one-tenth. It was also discovered that 90 to 95 per cent of rheumatic cases occurred before age 50; more than one-half before 30. Half the syphilitic cases occurred before 50; rarely before 30 or after 60. Eighty to 95 per cent of arteriosclerotic cases occurred after 50 years. Evidence was brought to bear furthermore on the difference that social status makes, on the course of these diseases and the question was raised, though it was not answered—indeed it is not yet answered—what are the conditions which bring the young to the clinics but keep the old away. Though it was then supposed, and is now well known, that a large older cardiac population exists, it was found, not in the clinics, but in the hospitals. With the growth in numbers of the aged population, the extent of the provision a community must provide has increased. The problem has become urgent, therefore, among the factors that enter social planning for the care of patients suffering from these ailments. In this study, Wyckoff and Lingg's appreciation of these issues was explicit. They have now become problems of great importance in medical statesmanship.

Of the opportunities which the conduct of his clinic suggested, Wyckoff took full advantage. He published papers on certain diseases of rheumatic origin, others on cases of arteriosclerosis or, as he sometimes called them, of senescence, and still others on pharmacology and treatment.

He could not, of course, escape profound interest in the arteriosclerotic form of cardiac disease, found in the latter decades, which has become numerically ever more important. The nature of the process responsible for this condition has engaged wide-spread but, I hesitate to say, inadequate interest. A defect in thinking, common when a direction of inquiry is young, is the optimistic belief that discoveries can be made rapidly without the need of long and painful dealing with and contemplation of simple phenomena. It is not difficult to find ample excuse for haste—problems cry for urgent solution; indeed they enlist our humane feelings so that delay seems inexcusable. But if successful thinking seems often to be a matter of brilliance, the long history of science exhibits a certain inexorability in the pace at which subjects and the comprehension of subjects unfold themselves. Something like this reflection must have lain in Wyckoff's mind when he thought of arteriosclerotic heart disease. In an address at the College of Physicians in Philadelphia, he reviewed the multitude of facts and half-facts, theories and vague suppositions in which the literature of this subject abounds. In the end he brushed them reluctantly aside and gave this as his belief:

"Many of the questions which we wish to answer could be answered today if the thousands of careful observations made in the various clinics in this city on patients having arteriosclerosis had been collected in a co-ordinated and uniform way, with the use of definite criteria, and if they had been placed upon a chart which would make them available for statistical study."

And he went on:

"It is my belief that the final answers to most of these questions will come from the careful study of patients in ambulatory clinics over long periods of time, where these patients are not only carefully studied, but where accurate and uniform data are obtained by every available method and, after being selected, scientifically analyzed."

Finally, he concluded:

"Physicians often marvel at the time and patience which a laboratory investigator expends in the development of a proper laboratory technique. Our work—that is, properly co-ordinated clinical and laboratory investigation in chronic disease—demands a technique which is surely as difficult to perfect and the development of which takes years." [14]

Not the least of Wyckoff's qualities was the penetratingness of his insight. He admired, perhaps extravagantly, the development of techniques for analyzing complex situations, we often call them laboratory studies, but his view was sufficiently spacious to understand that not methods, but subjects, form the objective of scientific enterprise. He was not taken in by the multitude and intricacy of experiments when they failed to elucidate the major problem, the question at issue.

When he came to collect his thoughts on the treatment of arteriosclerosis a little later in 1933, he had the courage to write:

"At present no evidence exists that there is any specific mode of therapy which can either cure or affect the progress of arteriosclerosis.

[14] "A Consideration of the Possibility of the Prevention of Arteriosclerotic Heart Disease." *Tr. College Physicians Philadelphia*, 1929, *51*, 95-108.

This statement is made after a fairly careful consideration of the subject and with a full realization that to make such a general statement is usually dangerous.

"The studies of the literature of the treatment of arteriosclerosis are confusing because of the lack of system in most discussions of the subject. Even among the best authorities treatment of cause, of symptoms, and of structural change is so jumbled as to make it difficult of analysis." [15]

It seems unnecessary to add anything to these statements.

Wyckoff had a quality which, unfortunately, had, in the exigencies of the life he led, little opportunity for development. The ability to make aphorisms, those genial and penetrating insights which are in essence, clinical sense, he possessed. With his humor and raciness he could not fail, sooner or later, to have become distinguished for a gift in this direction. I have been permitted to see the manuscript [16] of a paper, planned only a year after he took control of his clinic, and written in 1922 but never published, which deals with the functional capability of cardiac patients. Four paragraphs which I excerpt indicate this quality:

. . . in this series, patients once having had heart failure have little ability to do heavy work, and a great many of them are unable to do moderate work, though nearly all of them are able to do light work.

The ability of patients with auricular fibrillation to do work I do not believe can be determined, until after the patients have been thoroughly digitalized. After digitalization I believe that they react to occupation in direct proportion to the amount of good heart muscle they have.

I believe that this is a prognostic point of great importance: patients with auricular fibrillation who after full digitalization have insufficient reserve to do even light work have a very bad prognosis.

Women with organic heart disease do proportionately heavier work than do men. This we believe is not because of their greater physical

[15] "The Treatment of Arteriosclerosis." Chapter 20 in E. V. Cowdry, *Arteriosclerosis. A Survey of the Problem*, New York, 1933.

[16] This paper—called Dr. Wyckoff's First Paper—1922, deals with the functional capacity of 152 patients (male and female) registered in his clinic before June 15, 1920.

ability but because of the greater difficulty women over the age of thirty have in changing or modifying their vocations.

Stimulated by the success of the New York Heart Association and moved by a comparable situation in the nation, under the leadership of a group in New York, physicians in various communities came to the conclusion that the time had arrived for founding a national association. It was clear that the functions of the New York and of the national associations could not be identical. In New York it was possible and desirable to conduct a demonstration on a large scale, to show how in actual operation, cardiac clinics should be organized, supervised, and co-ordinated as a single enterprise. In the nation that experience bore fruit but in a different form—the National Association undertook to teach and to spread information. It adopted the nomenclature and the criteria of our New York Heart Association, it utilized our methods of recording histories and of entering abnormal physical signs, it taught, through leaflets, what was new and of accepted value. It brought into being, under the inspiriting editorship of Dr. Conner, The American Heart Journal. In making plans for the realization of these activities, in foreseeing what services could be rendered, in devising the plan and scope of the national organization, Wyckoff played a leading role. Dr. H. M. Marvin, the Secretary of the American Heart Association has written to me that on 24th May, 1922, 46 physicians met in St. Louis to discuss the possibility of forming a National Heart Association. The other members from New York were Alexander Lambert, Robert H. Halsey, Louis F. Bishop, Cary Eggleston, Harold E. B. Pardee, Haven Emerson. The certificate of incorporation was signed on 14th March, 1924. Wyckoff was not one of the 15 incorporators but was nevertheless deeply interested in the formation of the Association. Later he became a Director, a member of the Executive Committee for some years, and President for 2 years. Marvin writes: [17]

I can speak only in a very general way about his views concerning the policies which the Association should adopt. During the years that we

[17] January 13, 1938.

were fellow members of the Executive Committee, I believe it true to say that he had greater influence than any other one member of that Committee, with the possible exception of Dr. Conner. I believe this was not due to the warm affection that he inspired in all of us but rather to the fact that his advice and his views always seemed wise and right. For years he was a sort of unofficial liaison officer between the New York and American Heart Associations, and he always emphasized the importance of a close and friendly co-operation between these two groups. He was eager that the American Heart Association should render every possible educational help to practicing physicians, and it is Dr. Maynard's belief that he regarded the education of physicians as more important than education of lay people. He was heartily in favor of every attempt which aimed at making the Association a more truly national body in its representation and activities. As Chairman of the Reference Committee, he was largely responsible for the formulation of a program for the Association, which was formally adopted a few years ago and which perhaps indicates his ideas better than anything I can write. . . . In the seven or eight years preceding his death, I think that no important action of any sort was taken by the Executive Committee or Board of Directors without his active participation or at least his knowledge and advice. In the discussions that often occurred in committee meetings, I was always deeply impressed by his sanity, his wisdom, and his unfailing tolerance. Often (as in matters relating to the New York Heart Association or to groups and societies elsewhere in the country) he had direct and precise information which was of the greatest help.

Between the New York Heart Association and the National one Wyckoff acted, as Marvin says, as unofficial liaison officer. His experience, the soundness of his judgment, his good temper, were frequently called into play in helping to define the provinces within which the two associations could most naturally play their appointed roles. His labors bore admirable fruit—now, after a few years only, the methods of the two organizations are satisfactorily and adequately defined—friction has given place to co-operation —and mutual helpfulness has become established.

It is scarcely within my province to speak of Wyckoff's labors in the field of education. If I do so it is not to recount his exploits therein, but to let them serve to point out the catholicity, the soundness, and the straightforwardness of his judgment. His method of studying the value of previous academic training in preparation for medical education was especially noteworthy. The good college student, he showed, became the good medical student. And good meant, good in scholarship. He showed that when scholarship alone, without personal consideration, was used as a criterion for admission to medical study, failures in the medical school rapidly declined.[18] He understood, because of his fearlessness, how to appraise, how to gain insight into one of the most difficult problems which confront educators.

His presidental address to representatives of American medical colleges is, it seems to me, a model of wise, just, and communal views. Here he exhibited his strong social feeling with great good common sense. The glamor of shibboleths did not deceive him, nor did he mistake appearance for reality. The first business of a medical school he believed was to convey knowledge of diseases. No one understood better than he the responsibility which attached to the schools in providing for the advancement of learning. But it seemed incorrect to him, when teaching was inadequate, to devote much-wanted resources to research. He remembered how in Milton—the hungry sheep look up but are not fed. Contrariwise, he believed he saw better teaching and a closer relation of student and patient in schools said to be over-scientific; and the poorest clinical opportunities in the very schools where the greatest stress was laid on practical education. To make these observations and to be able to proclaim them without reproach is evidence of the enviable reputation for just views and for just feeling he had attained.

I come to the end of this account of the achievements of John Wyckoff with a feeling that I have done scant justice to his essential quality. Quality is necessarily fugitive. It is one of our grimmest realizations, how impossible it is to capture and to preserve it. Our experience of it, inevitably wearing thin through the years, we treasure nevertheless as an abiding possession. Wyckoff's out-

---

[18] "Relation of Collegiate to Medical
Student Scholarship." *Bull. Assn. Am.
M. Coll.*, 1927, 2, 1-16.

standing quality, I do believe, was of the heart—if that can be credited of a man so wise, so shrewd, so far-seeing. It was his heart dictated to him his attitude as a physician, made him aware of the dependence of patients upon his knowledge and power, made him sensitive to their need for understanding and sympathy. It never occurred to him to make distinctions in his personal attitude to men of high degree or of low. His abiding humanity drew both equally within the orbit of his compassionate regard. His rugged demeanor served but to heighten this effect. This quality of heart informed, I think, his every act, toward students, toward associates, toward colleagues. Whatever he did, in clinic, in hospital, in school, and in society, he did with an eye single to high attainment. And high attainment was conceived not for his personal, but for the general good. I end even as I began. There has passed from among us a man remarkable among men.

First published in *Bulletin of the History of Medicine* (Volume VI, Number 7, July, 1938).

The Meaning of Medical Research

A LECTURE TO THE LAITY

I N THE discussion which follows you may expect a description
of discoveries, dramatic and exciting perhaps; of new diseases
or an account of the discovery of mechanisms underlying diseases
already identified; of new drugs which cure, like sulphanilamide
or penicillin; of new operations which relieve or prevent serious
illness like arterial hypertension or mental agitation. I could en-
liven this report by such narratives, as for example the great new
insights which have resulted from studying the pituitary gland.
The investigation of this organ by Cushing who gave the forward
movement a great impetus and by many other very capable and
ingenious investigators, has resulted in the description of new ailments, has given point to the attempt to understand the interrelations of fluids and tissues and organs, in ways and to extents not
dreamed of ten years ago; has made available agents of real power
in adjusting defaulting or erring organs. Or in a sense less pathological and more physiological, I could describe how great has been
the increase in knowledge of the behavior of such important tissues
as muscle and nerve. But to speak of any one adequately would cost
all my time. There are other ample avenues, however, for spreading that sort of information. My task is both simpler and more
complicated. I am to speak of what research in medicine "means,"
what its nature is and what its purposes. And I take that to include an inquiry into its position in the complicated matrix of our
social structure.

The ultimate meaning or purpose of medical research is to rid
men of diseases, to protect them from maladies with which they
are threatened, to relieve them of discomforts once they are established. There are many diseases, differing in the degree of danger-
ousness, differing in nature, differing in geographic distribution.
There are illnesses of the existence of which we are aware and

which we investigate actively—others which, for various reasons, we ignore. The character of contemporary education is decisive in defining what can be attempted, having its sources and momentum partly in tradition and partly in response to current novelty. Researches are delayed because points of departure of importance are missed, medical scientists being unprepared to comprehend them and to pursue a possibility. Researches are sometimes hurried, wasteful, and erroneous, because of the faulty belief that current equipment is adequate to deal with particular problems. The status of public versus private scholarship is important—less important now when the whole situation of research begins to be better understood, and when private investigation in experimental science is recognized as being very much less practicable than formerly. Financial resources are now rarely sufficient to free private scholars so that they can pursue their own independent and uninfluenced conceptions, unimpeded by the restrictions which would be imposed upon them by administrators of public funds. Restrictions of any sort can unfortunately circumscribe the intellectual latitude which provides for personal vagary, for unorthodoxy, traits for the moment which may not be congenial in an academic environment. The reverse of this matter consists in a student's need, under any circumstances, private, semi-private or public, to persuade or convince an administrator to permit a research contrary to the administrant's inferior judgment. Failure to persuade can long retard advance. It can be a serious impasse. But still greater in importance, because inescapable, is the subtle and pervasive influence of current belief and opinion, current social need, and current economic situation which tend to limit or, perhaps better, which do not permit us to escape current intellectual tendencies. These are aspects of the intellectual life of which Hessen [1] and his followers have made us aware.[2]

[1] B. Hessen, "The Social and Economic Roots of Newton's *Principia*," in *Science at the Cross Roads,* papers presented to the International Congress of the History of Science and Technology, London, 1931, by delegates of the U. S. S. R., London, 1931.

[2] It is important to study the nature of social pressure, using this term in its widest sense, in the province of diseases. To apply this point of view is not strange to historians and students of social phenomena, but one not yet much employed in medical thinking. The

The meaning of medical research must regard these various social and personal aspects. It must regard also the nexus which exists between medical and other sciences. It must make an effort to understand likenesses and differences which characterize medicine in relation to those other sciences. It must analyze the situations, diseases and social pressures, to which energy is devoted and must describe the means, in men and facilities, which are available for carrying them out.

I propose to speak first of *what* we study; second of *how* we study it; third, of *who* does the studying; and finally, *for what reason* does the study take place.

While these far-reaching issues and conceptions are being canvassed certain situations in the world of diseases should first be described. It has already been suggested that diseases vary with time and place. It is not customary to study those diseases which do not exist, or which exist elsewhere, or which exist no longer. The impulse to study a certain disease or a given hygienic circumstance results from the danger or the damage which it causes. Epidemics of diseases like the black death or of poliomyelitis, or of influenza, or of cholera cannot safely be ignored. But not many of the resources of this community are devoted to yellow fever or kala-azar, or African sleeping sickness. If these diseases were, by their maritime introduction, to threaten the local population, a study of them would be inescapable.[3] They are studied though for several reasons; a general philanthropic motive; because, as in the opinion of Dr. Albert Schweitzer,[4] restitution

illustrations in this essay have been drawn chiefly from communicable diseases and from a few other maladies differently grouped. But the influence of nutrition as this has become better understood through investigations of the chemical processes on which nutrition depends; the influence of improved methods of agriculture; the influence of changing views more sympathetic to securing better food supplies for the less well circumstanced—all these have a bearing on problems of health. And this in turn has a bearing on the effort to understand the needs of the community as a whole and to find means of meeting them.

[3] This situation became actual during the war.

[4] Dr. Schweitzer is one of the remarkable men of our time. He is an Alsatian medical missionary in equa-

should be made to a people for the injury done them by others who have been exploiting them; because, to study them is imperative to preserve health along international trade routes. In any case local or temporary pressure of some sort is usually experienced or is exercised when a study is undertaken.

Of the diseases which we do study there are several kinds. It is of very great importance to understand that diseases cannot, all of them, be regarded as forming a coherent or a natural system. They can be grouped, as indeed they are, those of them which exhibit similar traits. The various groups have, superficially at least, little in common except that they transform the individuals whom they afflict.[5] Each group, on the other hand, exhibits phenomena which leave no or little doubt as to the relatedness of the members.

The center of gravity of interest in diseases has long, roughly for two generations, lain in *infectious* and *epidemic diseases*. To understand them, the sciences which needed to be and which were and are actively cultivated are bacteriology and parasitology. More recently diseases resulting from viruses, which are of far smaller dimensions than bacteria, have been added to the list. These diseases all depend on the invasion of animal and plant organisms by these agents. Parallel with bacteriology and parasitology, sciences roughly grouped as immunological have been developed, in which there have been studied the reactions, that is to say, the behavior of the hosts, plants and animals, which the infectious agents invade. Studies of invasion have gone further though than the study of individual hosts when under attack. A science of epidemiology has grown alongside the other sciences, to study the conditions in which societies of animals, plants and men chance to become suitable for invasion by infecting agents. The

torial Africa, a great organist. He has written an authoritative life of J. S. Bach.

[5] A disease is not an "entity" which takes possession of a person. A person affected becomes contrariwise a transformed organism. The organism is a physiological system so constituted as to dispose it to the exhibition of disease. The preparation may be constitutional or psychological or local—but the transformed organism is transformed by elements in addition to what is called an invader.

elements which are involved include external factors—race, climate, season, sunlight; and internal factors, the blood, the plasma, certain organs and tissues, and hereditary predisposition. To cope with invasions, efforts in various directions have sedulously been made—with sera, which utilize the forces that animal bodies themselves prepare for their protection; with chemicals, like salvarsan, like optochin, like arsphenamine, the sulpha drugs—all synthetized with the utmost chemical skill; with penicillin and other similar agents, with natural pharmacal agents, chaulmoogra oil, quinine, salicylates. These are, in a sense, beginnings, the successes of which point to the fact that the way of thinking about such problems as they represent, is sound and therefore encouraging. Much more is expected from such efforts. Indeed these are not more than auspicious beginnings.

A point of importance, later to be referred to, is that the successes, still in many instances not more than partial, have been attained by searching below the surface of appearances to gain information on the mechanism on which these diseases depend. Invaders and reactions—with this kind of knowledge as a background, substances of many sorts have been sought, to oppose the action of the invaders. Here are the rudiments, I may mention in passing, of analytical procedures. They represent something new in the study of diseases. Compared to the amount of energy which has been expended, the success so far achieved has, quite obviously, been extraordinary.

Infectious or contagious or epidemic diseases have often been characterized as acute. Acute means two things—that individuals are seized suddenly with disability, a matter of hours or minutes; and also that their duration is usually brief—though there are numerous exceptions, as tuberculosis, syphilis, and leprosy.

But there are long-drawn-out ailments, often called *chronic*, which fall into two great groups. Certain ones occur at all ages, like pernicious anemia or diabetes mellitus. But there are others which befall older persons exclusively. I designate these "ailments" and not diseases, nor yet degenerative—two words often applied to them which I prefer not to use for reasons which I hope later to develop.

To distinguish diseases merely according to their duration is a crude conception. But to do so has a use, for the time being. Chronic has usually been intended to signify long-drawn-out. Roughly, chronic and long-drawn-out mean the same thing. From the point of view of patients and their families, duration is important; and from that of administrators concerned with the public health the distinction is essential. Actually what is involved is the rate at which the processes, in different maladies, the morbid mechanisms, advance. Chronic diseases or long-drawn-out maladies include a wide range of complaints. Their duration is to be estimated, naturally, from their beginning to their termination, uninfluenced, in order to be accurate, when such examples are available, by treatment. The group is multiform—there are, for example, the diseases of the blood-forming organs—pernicious anemia, leukemia, thrombocytopenia; there is cancer; there is tuberculosis; there are the deformities of the joints; there are cardiac and arterial derangements; there are the defects which result from insufficience or malfunction of the glands of internal secretion—of the hormones in short; there are diseases of the nervous system. It has been customary to divide diseases into three, or perhaps better two, main groups as I am doing; bacteriological and physiological. In both, but in the latter especially, physical and chemical techniques are employed in studying them. Chronic diseases fall into both groups. These categories require in certain instances to be stretched fairly wide, in order to include all the varieties. But they will serve for this discussion, especially if, in studying bacterial diseases, the behavior of the host, immunology, is included; and if in the physiological ones, anatomical defects and malformations.

It is illuminating, I think, to reflect that the whole discipline of medicine, as now constituted, deals with many kinds of conditions and that they fall roughly into the categories that have been indicated. Of chief moment is that the classification, though rough, is descriptive enough to indicate that there are groups sufficiently well characterized so that they can be recognized and that, through this possibility, study is facilitated, perhaps made possible.

Now it is generally understood and indeed it must be obvious

that when a malady or for that matter any other natural phe
nomenon begins to be *analyzed* (analysis being the method essen
tial to experimental research) very soon a level of organizatio
is reached, less complex than the native state of a whole plant o
animal, the study of which requires recourse to a chemical labora
tory. This is owing to the fact that biological mechanisms, whe
the attempt is made to view them "working," can be made t
break down promptly into recognizable chemical processes. I
physiological diseases, especially those of the heart and arteries, i
parallel fashion, a structural stage is soon reached when mechani
cal and physical appliances are needed to help in understandin
what is going on. To turn to chemistry, to mechanics, to physics
is to turn not so much to fundamental things as to machinery th
function of which is to aid in the effort to understand more com
plex, directly observable behaviors. These disciplines to which on
turns—physics, chemistry, immunology—provide the technique
which are used to analyze, to reduce to simpler, more easily under
standable mechanisms, the surface appearance of maladies. Th
fact that this is the situation in research in diseases constitutes
dilemma. To this problem it will be necessary to return.

I have referred to *two kinds of chronic diseases*—one whic
can occur at any age and one which is characteristic of the age
Those diseases characteristic of the *aged* require especial descrip
tion because, though they are not new, they are beginning t
take on new significance. We grow older, all of us. As is we
known, in the course of doing so we fall subject predominantl
to several distinct kinds of disabilities. I pass over cancer; its natur
and its ravages are in everyone's mind. But what happens to th
heart, the arteries and the kidneys, has been less clearly appreciate
I do not wish to discuss all the possibilities, all the theories. On
theory ought I think to be more fully described. In the sense th
everybody ages, aging has come to be looked upon as a natur
phenomenon—natural, as differing from accident or from chanc
Since everyone ages, aging is correctly or incorrectly anticipate
and the separate phenomena of aging are looked upon as predict
ble. This has been a subject of very active research in recer

years. And the objectives in such researches have been twofold; first, to ascertain as precisely as possible a description of what actually takes place and second, to discover what mechanisms are at work to bring about the results observed.

I single out the arteries for more detailed description. That the arteries change is now universally known, especially the great artery of the body, the aorta. What is less well known is that the smaller ones do also. Arteries which have come in for marked attention in recent years are those of the heart—the coronary arteries. The walls of arteries may be thought of as having layers or coats, as do modern rubber garden hoses. In the coronary arteries, for example, the first detectable changes take place in the innermost layer. This includes an elastic membrane which splits in two and does so rather early in life—in the twenties. From then on, more and more changes take place. At fifty or sixty these changes are advanced and have been termed arteriosclerosis because the arteries feel hard. To one familiar with the succession of microscopic appearances, it is possible to tell their age, within a few years. Being able to do this is good evidence that there is nothing haphazard about the process. It may ultimately, when everything is known, be unnecessary, but it is not haphazard. How are these systematic changes brought about? And how, assuming that they develop systematically, can they be prevented or delayed? To answer these questions, guesses have been ventured since very early times and to explain them, serious, far-reaching researches have been undertaken. But so far there are no answers satisfactory to many scientists. Meanwhile the quest goes on, with intensifying earnestness. The problem, as I shall show presently, is urgent. What is true of the arteries of the heart is true of those of the brain. About other organs less is known. Progressive alterations, appropriate to each organ and tissue, go on throughout the body—beside the heart muscle, in the kidneys, in the liver—everywhere in short.

But changes in structure do not alone exhibit progressive alteration. Comparable ones can be observed also in the functioning of the body. The slow and gradual rise with age which the blood pressures exhibit is well known. Another striking one has, for example, recently been found in a secretion of the body. Here, it appears that ptyalin, the starch-splitting ferment of the saliva, decreases between twenty-five and eighty-one (these are averages) to one thirty-fourth, necessitating, it seems probable, a very striking readjustment in digestion and food requirements in the aged. More intimate still are changes in behavior of the muscle fibers of the heart. It has been shown in dogs, for example, that as the animals grow older, the ability of this tissue to utilize oxygen diminishes significantly. Finally, as in changes in structure and in function, so also, it appears, can changes in psychological performance be detected. Interest in this phase of growth has begun more recently, so that it would be rash to accept the results of preliminary studies. There can be little doubt though that this is a fruitful field for further investigation.[6]

Many regard it as an idle question, but it is one which should be put nevertheless—are processes so universal as are those identified with aging to be regarded as diseases? Diseases, at least those occurrences which are designated diseases, are not constant; they wax and wane; new ones occur; old ones vanish; they are unlooked for; they are recovered from. Of the changes which accompany aging, none of these characteristics can be predicated. It seems better to weigh the question of the nature of this process of aging a while longer, before coming to a decision on its nature. Two ways of thinking are possible—that aging is an accident which can be prevented; or that it is not an accident and that, as the body increases in bulk and by so doing is said to grow, parallel changes are taking place within the body, in its most intimate recesses. These changes accompany growth and may themselves be regarded as taking part in and perhaps constituting the phenomena of growth. They keep on even when bulk ceases to increase. In this sense the body grows continuously. Changes, called differentiation, take place in all parts, the form of change

---

[6] This reference to psychological matters is brief because I am depending on other phases of this problem for illustration. But the place in human nature and in diseases which psychological deviations occupy can scarcely be over-emphasized. I am at one with those who wish to understand organisms as wholes and to return from the wilderness into which the requirements of thought in the 17th Century naturally led us.

altering from stage to stage, that is to say from year to year, without break, until the final dissolution. This view urges that there is only one forward-moving process—not, first growth and then degeneration, but continuous progressive differentiation. And growth so understood is not an accident, it is not degeneration—and it is not disease.

These old ailments present a new challenge. To care for them is becoming a great burden, financially. Can anything be done to relieve the strain? Medical research, not yet very consciously, is struggling with the question. It has no settled answer. When such questions were first raised fifteen years ago, we were not yet ready to weigh them. Now the response may become, is indeed becoming, more intelligent. The old hospitals built for infectious diseases will no longer serve. In part they are improperly constructed for these purposes. And from the point of view of research, the new situation calls for new orientation, for institutions of a new type with different, expanded facilities for research. It is still inescapable that research in infectious diseases continue here and elsewhere. Here, because there is still tuberculosis, syphilis, poliomyelitis and other infections of the nervous system, rheumatic fever and influenza; elsewhere, in the tropics, because of diseases indigenous there, but perhaps transplantable here. But since the dawn of that era in which we have spent our lives, the emphasis has been almost exclusively on diseases of this kind. It would be incorrect to say that diseases longer drawn out at older ages had been neglected—cancer for example or cardiac diseases. But it is certain that in comparison with infectious diseases, they have been much less cared for and studied. The great desideratum now is, to turn increasing attention to these conditions. If they were better understood, it might become possible to manage them better. If they were better treated, expensive care in homes and in institutions might be less necessary; if they were less expensively treated, the burden of taxation might diminish. The net result would accrue vastly to the sufferers themselves—in increased health, in greater freedom spent outside of institutions, in greater economic self-sufficiency. Psychologically, the lives of older men and women might be re-made if we learned how to make them self-sufficient

to a degree impossible now, through a new orientation to employment, utilizing opportunities for activity appropriate to the aged.
Embedded in the matrix of current society, no better fate is provided for them or envisaged than progressive deterioration.

I have been speaking of *what* we study. I come now to speak
of *how* we do so. After long reflection and practical experience
there has come to be general comprehension of the purposes and
methods of the sciences in general. By the same token, a similar
statement can be made of medical science. But in some subtle way
there is tacit agreement that the two are in essence somehow different. Whether they are, depends I think upon the aspect from
which this judgment is made. They do not differ, there would
be general agreement, in attitude to natural phenomena; nor do
they differ in the seriousness with which the problems of diseases
are studied; nor do they differ in the methods which both, or all
use. To recognize and to point out the remaining differences is
not invidious; no more is intended than to understand a complicated situation.

Two suggest themselves—first, one having to do with the
nature of the subject matter; and second, one having to do with
the circumstances conditioning the activities of students of disease.
The former, different in subject matter, has, I venture to believe, a certain validity; [7] the second, I think, not. To begin with,
though it is not my intention to become involved merely in words
it is well to make clear the meaning I ascribe to certain terms.

Science, very briefly, as I have been saying, is a way of looking
at nature, exactly, in so far as that is possible. Two elements are
involved—the natural phenomena themselves, and a way of
looking.

[7] It is perhaps a superficial experience but one to which large numbers
of persons are sensitive, that in a very
general sense, diseases are ugly, repel-
lent, offensive. These are not qualities
which characterize phenomena studied in
other sciences. The reverse may be and
often is true. It is of course a fact that
to many men, perhaps especially to
physicians, this aspect of diseases is
without meaning. It may be that to
them the very fact of ugliness has the
value of attraction. Nor need this be regarded as odd. The last word on the
subject of ugliness has not been uttered
—respecting sight, sound, or form.

Research is science's way of looking. Research is procedure. Research represents the effort men make to increase their comprehension. To discover what is true about anything is an arduous undertaking because, at the outset, so many things seem possibly correct. That is why research is an adventure.

The object of the whole enterprise is to *describe* nature.[8] At first it seems wise, at all event it seems to have been universally customary, to describe natural phenomena so as to group them. That makes description easier because there result fewer descriptions. Classification is what this phase of the undertaking is called. Sometimes, especially in our day, there lurks, unfortunately, something invidious in the remark that an investigator is merely "describing." Descriptions must naturally be exact. Exactness can in fact be exhibited, purely and deliberately, without quantitative expression, in descriptions of things as they occur in nature, rough and in the whole. Men who have carried on this phase of natural inquiry have been known as naturalists or, at a stage more organized, more complicated, systematists. Hippocrates, Pliny, Albertus Magnus, Linnaeus, Sydenham, Darwin, Lyell, Audubon, Wheeler, form such a group. Their very names are proof that nothing derogatory attaches to their interests or their methods. Without labors like theirs, there can be no natural science. Without them we should be talking of phoenixes, unicorns and griffins. It is evidence of the literalness of the culture of the Greeks that, unlike Egyptians or Orientals, they entered little into nature faking. The objects of interest to scientists have been natural objects. Later —and later may be taken to have a chronological meaning, though it may have also a logical one—when the *experimental era* began in its modern form, reliance came to be placed, not by any means exclusively but accompanied by a certain glamor which obscured the relative value among methods, on the experimental method.

[8] There are those to whom action appears a more impressive and compelling motive than description. The object of the enterprise would then be to accomplish an end. But to accomplish an end without comprehending the machine is scarcely reasonable. The difference is essential but it may also be a difference in emphasis. If astronomy began in the interests of action, it has remained a means to satisfy mere curiosity; or—is it perhaps to return to its original function?

A powerful agent for extending knowledge became available. The experimental method involves the conception that comprehension of a thing, of a phenomenon, can be furthered powerfully by dissecting it, by pulling it apart, by measuring and by weighing and by counting.[9] I need not dwell on, what is universally known, the extraordinary and unbelievable success of the method. By it Galilei, Harvey, Newton, Young, Lavoisier, their modern equally great successors and a host of followers have enriched modern thought, modern knowledge and modern life.

When the experimental era began in its current form, the temptation was great to believe that, once the parts were known, the whole would be comprehended. It was another way of thinking that the whole is equal to the sum of the parts. But doubt began to be entertained that matters were not so simple. It was the same situation that confronted the King's horses and the King's men when they tried, after his fall, to put Humpty Dumpty together again. Because they failed and because the conviction is current and widespread that they cannot succeed, the idea has been put forward by S. Alexander, Lloyd Morgan, A. N. Whitehead and General Smuts that, in putting things together again after they have been taken apart, something new emerges, something not in the constituent elements. It is, to use a crude example, as if $2 + 2$ equal more than 4, because something not in the synthesizer's hands, or mind, entered into the new substance or new situation. The doctrine that something new occurs has come to be known as "emergent evolution." In speaking of analysis and synthesis it is unnecessary to lay undue emphasis on the imperfections of the methods, but it is desirable to be alive to their existence so as to anticipate the disappointments which otherwise are almost inescapable. There have in point of fact been a goodly number. Leaving aside the emergence of new qualities, a phase after all of synthesis, the delays which have taken place in finding the cures of infectious diseases, like tuberculosis, like typhoid fever,

[9] It needs scarcely to be pointed out that what is called synthesis, as in the preparation of chemical substances, dyes, for example; or aromatic compounds; or in metallurgy when new alloys are made; or in technical procedures or advances in general, is an extension merely of the analytical process.

like poliomyelitis, even after the discovery and identification of the agents that help to occasion them, are known to everybody.

The whole adventure, classification and analysis, is science. Science, I have said, has two aspects, the natural phenomena themselves and a way of looking. Of the way of looking enough has been said. Of the natural phenomena a significant difference exists between medical and other natural sciences. To this difference I wished to direct attention. The point that needs weighing is the character of *enduring interest* which attaches to other natural sciences and to a much slighter extent, the medical ones. Consider such interests as the origin of species, the movements of astronomical systems, matter, heat, electricity, the formation of the earth, light, heredity. These are inquiries as little influenced as may be by time and place. There was never a time when they did not engage serious intellectual attention; they do so now; there is good reason to believe they will continue to do so. These phenomena awoke and continue to awake enduring interests because they are enduring objects.

Turn in the same sense to the significance of diseases. I have been dwelling on enduringness in interest in the objects studied in the natural sciences because these are themselves enduring. Now diseases, whether of plants or of animals, no matter what their nature, are something extra.[10] They are occurrences which, in subtle or coarse ways, change the usual behavior of living things. They become something else. The organisms are said to suffer— hence the use of the word, in the British sense, pathology. Beside being something extra, their existence is not necessarily permanent. They change with time, they change with locality. The sweating sickness is gone. How long poliomyelitis may have existed is not

[10] I mean by extra—not anticipated among "healthy" persons. I do not mean that process "a" is added to organism "b" and that a + b when conjoined constitute a disease. In this sense "a" would be what has been called an entity—an "ens." That is far from my meaning. "Extra" describes the whole transformed organism, exhibiting phenomena not counted on as occurring in health. Health is a statistical conception from which a diseased organism is something quite different from a mere deviation. This subject is more fully discussed in the essay "Physiology and Medicine" in *Medicine, Science and Art: Studies in Interrelations,* Univ. Chicago Press, 1931, p. 164.

known. It came; it may go. Diseases devastating in the tropics do not exist in the temperate zones. In other cases, like rheumatic fever, the reverse may be true. Any infectious disease may continue to turn out to be a transient sojourner. By paying a necessary price, there are diseases of which we can be rid—syphilis for example, perhaps scarlet fever, no doubt a number of others. Diseases, furthermore, have no independent existence; they are recognized when they have transformed the nature of their hosts, plant or animal, temporarily or permanently.

If, as I have been surmising, enduringness is a characteristic of things which have become continuing objects of study in the natural sciences, it seems apparent that diseases do not partake of that quality. That is clearly the case with infectious diseases. Nor in all probability do chemical diseases, of which the deficiency states are examples, pellagra, pernicious anemia, rickets and scurvy.

Another group of diseases of great importance may be designated physiological. Physiology may be termed the study of the living behavior of an organism, differing from mere alteration in its structure. In the study of diseases, the physiology of an animal has importance because it occupies a place like the study of combustion in the mechanism of a steam engine. But a disease is not merely a quantitative change in physiology. A disease is something over and above and therefore different from this. The place of physiology in this scheme must be accurately defined, or I shall come to grief. Physiology undertakes an analysis in animals or plants which makes them going concerns. Since they themselves, being species, are enduring, so are the mechanisms on which their lives depend, as for instance the circulation, reproduction, digestion. These mechanisms are neither temporary nor local. They can go out of order. When they do, these physiological derangements are usually called diseases. Eclampsia is an example, or perhaps a certain variety of arterial hypertension, or fibrillation of the auricles of the heart, or psychogenic hyperthyroidism. A special case is that of senescence—the aging process through which we all pass. Enduringness itself is a relative term. Species and perhaps even whole genera come and go. The distinction I have drawn is naturally not quite clear-cut. Evolution and the disappearance of species and genera see to that. But there is enough background to occasion social consequences of great importance to the position of medicine.[11]

I wish now to examine the use of another word—"empiricism." When a certain amount of animadversion is intended in the use of the word, the adjective "crude" is sometimes prefixed. This phrase "crude empiricism" has been used especially with reference to the study of diseases, the assumption being that the study of diseases is something apart, in fact, from other studies of natural phenomena—something perhaps a little backward. On more careful reflection it becomes clear that "crude empiricism" is a phrase applicable to a level of discovery at which, what is called "thinking" has not been much employed or cannot be, in the absence of sensitive awareness or in the existing state of knowledge. Now, when what is called "crude empiricism" is exhibited the analysis of the subject matter under investigation is relatively in a raw state and the means which are used to analyze it are not, in comparison with those used elsewhere, in some other discipline, of a sort which deserves to be called refined. An example in medicine is the use of quinine in malaria before either the nature of malaria or the composition of quinine was known. The use of mercury in syphilis is another example, or of digitalis in dropsy. In physical science on the other hand, telephony and the nature of electricity, where means and ends are nicely adjusted, though a very rough analogue, may serve as example. The form in which I have stated this situation suggests its meaning. When something is done or some modification of a system is undertaken, as in the examples

[11] And yet, some contributions to general knowledge result from the study of ephemeral phenomena or from acquaint with transient experience. Contributions so derived can, no doubt, exert significant influence in developing insights, conceptions and procedures which come much later to fruition. Broad intellectual streams can originate in obscure rills. But there remains nevertheless a value which enduringness, as a method of characterization, possesses. Even so, as a characteristic, it is unnecessary to assume that it has more than relative value. Were diseases dependent on a relation to bacteria wholly to disappear, bacteriology, for example, having received its great stimulus from this association, may remain nevertheless an important interest because of the growing place it is coming to occupy in agriculture and elsewhere.

just given, it is in the natural, organized state of the material, the crude, native state, in which the operation is performed. There exists no guide, furthermore, to suggest what form the interference should take. If malaria is not known to be protozoal in origin, or if it is unknown that the infecting agent is susceptible to quinine, but a therapeutic attempt is made, none-the-less—that attempt is empirical and may be termed crude. The attempt should, naturally, be made. If the object is to understand—anything whatever, a beginning must be, indeed it usually is, made. Once a beginning is made, successive efforts at understanding, if on the road to success, become less and less "crude." In the case of matter, electricity, energy, methods of analysis have now become so refined that it is evident how long a distance has been traveled from rubbing cat's fur on amber (electron) merely to obtain a spectacular effect. The more purposefully we analyze, the further investigation becomes removed from crudity. Because analysis takes place in successive simple stages; because, covering the heart of a phenomenon there are layers, like the petals covering the heart of an artichoke which need to be penetrated or removed, Sherrington was moved to say behind each mechanism is hidden another mechanism. That is the way an experimenter must look at the world. Obviously the metaphor of the artichoke is imperfect for there is a last layer of small leaves, apparently confused in arrangement, and then the heart. But in nature, who knows when the last petal has been plucked and the heart of a natural process uncovered? There is a chance here (and the man who knows how to take it is the artist in science) that to discover *an* object, it is unnecessary—it may in fact be destructive, to go further than a certain point—the point being the emergent level for which search, the investigation, was undertaken. Protection against pneumonia will, by way of illustration, be solved far short of the atomic level. If the appropriate level is passed, the nature of the thing sought eludes one's grasp. Hawthorne's story of the birthmark and beauty tells the story of the devastation wrought by a perfectionist.

Whether knowledge is empirical depends often on the standpoint of the critic. A molecule, a protein molecule, may seem very refined in comparison with a man, but to an electron it looks enormously complex. The whole business is relative.

The point about empiricism and crudeness requires no further laboring. It must be apparent that at the beginning nothing else than crudeness is possible. Later on, though insight may have been gained, the term may still be applicable. Were the process of causation simple, as it is not, it would be possible to prescribe how a situation must be analyzed and possible to prophesy the results. There is little confidence nowadays that that can often be the case. Further understanding depends therefore on trial and error in the choice of analytical techniques. Since that is all but inescapable all scientific analysis is crude and all knowledge empirical. The only point of view from which empirical knowledge is less crude depends on the amount of relevant research that has succeeded. Much has become known about malaria and syphilis, about quinine and mercury, about dropsy and digitalis, about energy and electrons. But to him who must choose the *next* step, the situation contains elements of crudity which he recognizes as not far removed from that of that predecessor of his who took the adventurous *first* step. So long as there are further steps there is adventure and so long as there is adventure there is crudity. Otherwise research would be a commonplace procession along the avenues of the known. Bohr would be the last to underestimate Democritus.

He who tells us we must halt an inquiry until analysis has proceeded further must be certain of a number of matters around which this discussion has taken place. He must believe that further analysis of a complex situation is rewarding. A chemist preparing therapeutic agents will appreciate this point. Suppose it were optochin he had prepared and were told that too frequently giving his preparation caused blindness. Against pneumococci his agent worked admirably—destroying them was his original object. To perfect his agent and to safeguard a patient against unexpected, unfortunate consequences, what must he do? Must he search for other substances, similar in structure, must he try a quite different group of agents, or must he, by analyzing optochin further, hope to discover what is offending in the structure of his drug so that it may escape exerting a destructive influence upon human eyes?

Quinine and quinidine afford another example. The auricles, the entrance chambers of the hearts of human beings and other animals, often lose their custom of orderly contraction and do what we call fibrillate—a state in which they act in a very disorderly fashion. A sufferer from this disorder once noticed that frequently when he took quinine, the normal behavior of his heart was restored. He narrated his experience to his physician in Vienna, Professor Wenckebach. Professor Wenckebach sought to repeat his patient's attempts but met with scant success—and told this story in one of his treatises. It occurred to another physician—Frey—to try more or less systematically other chemical substances with which quinine is related. At this point it is valuable to consider certain personal matters. Was that a rational procedure of Frey's— was there good reason to think other quinine-like substances would work better than quinine? If so, which one and how related to quinine? Or should he explore other substances—not quinine but substances belonging to that series? Or should he attempt to build up quinine into a drug more complex? Or should he break it down to find what in quinine actually worked in Professor Wenckebach's patient—purify the drug in short? Or should he look for a substance which, in Professor Wenckebach's patient, aided quinine but was absent in his own? Or did his own patient harbor a substance which interfered with the action of quinine? All these were possibilities. A complete account of what Frey did is unknown— it usually is. He may have tried none of these or many. He had a single guide only. He was told quinine worked in a *single* person.

We were discussing levels of organization. The only point of immediate concern is whether he should have analyzed further to find a simpler substance. It may be, he should have done so, for what he did has not been wholly effective. What Frey did was to explore other drugs having organizations like quinine sulphate. He found in the group a substance which worked 60 per cent of the time, quinidine sulphate, identical with quinine sulphate except for its action on polarized light. This was turned left

—quinine turns it to the right. The structural formula symbolizes the difference; the two are written as mirror images of each other. Frey undertook no further analytical procedures. Success, only partial, it is true, was achieved on the same level of organization as before. There was no way of knowing beforehand either that quinidine would work when quinine would not, nor that quinidine would work only two-thirds of the time. It was not known, it is not known now, what causal relation is essential in this reaction. It is probably not yet profitable to search for it.[12]

It is in the nature of things that students of any phenomenon must have first-hand knowledge of that phenomenon itself. For simple description, first-hand acquaintance is all that is requisite. For analysis it is essential in addition, to possess knowledge of the art and practice of appropriate forms of analysis. There is no fundamental difference in the character of these procedures for students of diseases and for other natural scientists. Nor is there a difference in the operations which the mind undertakes. The intellectual powers which are appropriate are the same, whether the object of study is a disease or an electron. The physical methods employed in laboratories naturally differ and must especially be adapted to the objectives and material being analyzed. But the mind proceeds always in the same way; it knows how to perform a few tricks only and these few it employs indifferently wherever it has use for them. The mind measures, indifferent to the reason for doing so, length or volume or frequency. Its behavior remains always the same irrespective of the tools it uses—it describes, it classifies, it dissects. Experience must necessarily come first and then the analysis of that experience, whatever the object.

But a difference exists nevertheless. The practice of medicine is an ancient calling. It is as intricate as it is ancient. To practice it is one of the nicest of the arts. Its practitioners have been in the habit of serving in many social capacities. These have been so absorbing that until almost contemporary time neither leisure nor opportunity nor desire existed to proceed beyond simple descrip-

[12] I am of course aware that I am raising the issue raised by Hume. I am not certain whether this is not the illustration that shows how a rational attempt to arrive at "cause" breaks down.

tion. To undertake experimental, analytical research has but recently begun. But now the gap between practice and analyzing is by way of being bridged. The existence of the gap can no longer be ignored. At the same time too much has been made of its deterring effect—in my judgment much too much. When students were inadequately, or not at all trained for research, more emphasis was placed on the exclusive demands of practice than now. Much has changed, not least the estimate placed on traditional knowledge and on practical legerdemain, though medical opinion still insists upon transmitting a great deal of this in formal education. Two types of persons interested in diseases are now emerging, one interested in advancing knowledge about them, and the other in treating them. The difference is similar to the difference between engineers and physicists. Physicians who wish to learn how to analyze, can do so now—and do so to very useful purpose. But the gap, the difficulty I have mentioned, persists. It is real and it is important. Who would suppose, for example, that Graves' disease (exophathalmic goiter), in order properly to be comprehended requires knowledge of physiological occurrences and chemical processes, obviously not necessarily within the competent knowledge of conscientious practitioners of medicine? Or in the kind of cardiac affection common in older individuals, who would require of practitioners insight into and knowledge of the control of the most intimate behavior of muscle fibers? And not only that, but knowledge of what underlies the behavior of those muscle fibers and their ability to carry on work. I have spoken of other difficulties which beset physicians, but here is a major one—the gap between two kinds of competence. To treat what is so obviously wrong, he must have learned, in physiology and physics and chemistry, what a man can learn only, if he learn it at all, as the result of the expenditure of all his energy. To carry on both, research and practice, in these circumstances, was at an impasse. For twenty-five years and more the effort has been made to bridge this gap by providing opportunity for a few physicians at least, to free themselves from the demands of practice. The divorce of research from demands so continuously absorbing has accomplished noteworthy results. Whether the divorce is adequate has not, I think, received sufficient scrutiny—nor whether there should be one.

Opportunity for research has now been gained and a certain amount of irrelevant information has been left at the wayside. Physicians have bettered their chance to observe the phenomena of diseases. They have better facilities now through their intimate contact with patients and their ailments, to ferret out the meaning of what they observe. No one else has access to that knowledge. Having that knowledge and the requisite training, physicians, specially chosen, are moving into position to solve relevant problems of diseases. It would be idle to underrate the difficulties. These do not so much consist in translating problems from bedside to laboratory as from translating one pattern of knowledge with its technical (clinical) apparatus to another quite different pattern with equally exacting, if not more complicated, technical (chemical and mechanical) apparatus. To recognize, for example, a cardiac disease, to think of its origin, to study its future, is obviously a different enterprise from a search for the mechanism of the contraction of muscle on which a person's or a patient's physical activity depends. For that search involves far away knowledge of proteins and the part they play in the complex structure and contraction of muscle. Other illustrations may be chosen— syphilis, for example, its dependence on a microorganism—a spirochete—and the susceptibility of spirochetes to poisoning by arsenical and other compounds. Or still another, diabetes mellitus, depending essentially on destruction or malfunction of the islands of Langerhans in the pancreas and the correction of this condition with a substance extracted from these islands.

This discussion and these illustrations should suffice to define a peculiar situation in medical science. I have already spoken of one special characteristic—the absence of "enduringness" and of universality exhibited by diseases. I have now illustrated the wide interval stretching between diseased persons, diseases as clinical appearances, and the cumbersome methods necessary in studying them. The inescapable combination of (a) clinical methods which may not do violence to patients demanding very exact, time-consuming training, with (b) analytical procedures explains how the position of medical science has come to be different from that in other sciences. In this complicated situation the intellectual position of medical scientists is often looked upon as differing from that of other scientists.

It is clearly impossible to exaggerate the importance of treatment. The motives which have brought great funds into existence to facilitate study have not, except in connection with great dangers, arisen from general public interest. The year 1776 was remarkable, aside from having witnessed the signature of the Declaration of Independence, for the effort Johann Peter Frank (see page 126) made, on behalf of the Archbishop of Speyer, to gather information on a social, political, or at all events on a grand scale, concerning the health of a population, so as to make this more secure. That enterprise began an epoch. Usually, it has been the illness of a friend or a member of a family that has stimulated the aroused interest of private philanthropists. The universities have had no available funds. Government has taken a minimum interest only.[18]

Once, when I defined medicine as the study of *diseases*, Doctor Thayer objected vigorously because in his judgment, joined inseparably to the study of diseases, was the need to get on with the business of curing diseases. The term medicine, he thought, included both. Obviously a term can mean whatever we say that it does. There is no reason against the use of the term "medicine" in the manner on which Dr. Thayer insisted. It is preferable though, I think, not to make the meaning of terms too inclusive; that is a way of obscuring the variety of aspects which a situation can be made to disclose. It is undoubted, indeed in the world of medicine the notion is widespread, that to search out the nature of diseases is itself a major obligation. But there is no doubt that the notion of curing diseases is universally believed to be a function of physicians. There should indeed be no doubt that this is so. The function of "medicine" to concern itself with the *cure* of diseases is so deeply embedded in both public and professional minds

[18] Evidence for this view is supplied by the attempt now being made to create a National Research Foundation in the United States.

that there have been periods of impatience with the conception that curing is difficult and complicated and with those who have insisted on education more or less elaborate for men whose office it might become to search out cures. Joining the search for knowledge of diseases with curing diseases has, I think, tended to obscure the problems presented by both. It is not without importance to point out that to make cures and to practice medicine provides, within properly defined limits, for a dispersed kind of activity not encountered in other disciplines.

Cures are of two kinds—we have depended on what I have been calling "crude" empiricism for one of them. Here there is no need for the refinement of analytical procedures. Even if agents are not rationally related to complaints they should be used if they succeed to mitigate them. Such agents do turn up, as digitalis in the case of dropsy, suggested by the Shropshire housewife who interested the co-operative Dr. Withering in her experiences; or when, owing to faith in the providence of God, the notion is entertained that where diseases occur, there in close proximity are their cures to be found—as salicylic acid (the willow) in the case of rheumatic fever.

The other kind of cure relies on nothing so simple, nothing so fortuitous. In this case cures are conceived possible because of a belief that there exists something in a morbid condition, central to it, a knowledge of which would further the possibility of cure, as the presence of microorganisms in typhoid fever; or of toxins in diphtheria; or of excess activity of an organ, as in thyroid hyperactivity; or deficiency in a secretion, as in pernicious anemia; or defect or destruction in tissues or organs, exerting either immediate or remote consequences, as the effect on the heart in beri-beri, or of the late result, again on the heart, of rheumatic fever; or, pursuit, perhaps vain, in the irrational footsteps of Ponce de Leon, of substances which neutralize the action of agents that make the body age.

But how are such substances to be found? They are actually and feverishly being sought. The sciences of chemotherapy, physico-therapy, immunology, pharmacology, the founding of institutes for the study of cancer and for this, that or the other, are evidence of the liveliness of the quest. Sometimes the direction of research is simple enough—the agents being already well known; in the case of hemolytic streptococcus infections, sulphanilamide, and now penicillin and its allies; in tetanus, tetanus antitoxin; in the failure of cardiac muscle, digitalis. But in the case of cancer the situation is different. In this disease neither cause nor cure is known. There may not, in fact, be a single disease, cancer, but a number having several characteristics in common. Shall the search be for an agent to combat a virus or some other substance or for the correction of a constitutional arrangement responsible for the licentious growth? The direction which the search is to take is often the subject of sharp cleavages of opinion. The single subject, cancer, illustrates how in the process of analysis, talents, equipments, trainings of different forms are serviceable. If you believe cancer is caused by a virus you want men to search for this who are perhaps differently endowed and certainly differently equipped from men who believe the solution of this problem lies in discovering a chemical substance to be neutralized, responsible for its origin or development.

Since there is here no desire to rely on haphazard, no other guide but reason is available. But reason must operate in the domain of causation and its tool is argument informed by insight or experience in action. Now, as has long been evident, reason alone is inadequate. The procedure though is the use of reason to limit the area of investigation so that then, within narrow, indeed within the narrowest framework possible, systematic trial and error can be attempted. If science is empiric, somehow experience provides it with a pattern. That is Aristotelian. Here is the appointed region for the display of scholarship, ingenuity, resource. What the issue is, in seeking the cause or cure of cancer, no one now, I presume, would be bold enough to declare. It is a fortunate circumstance that men of many minds, everywhere, are engaged in this search. But the point to be made is that once the method of crude empiricism is abandoned, the alternative, which is analysis, requires technical education not at the disposal of everyone interested in a subject. The problem is the problem of the physician as scientist. Special training is the prerequisite price to be paid for analysis, and analysis is the consequence of the failure of the pursuit of the obvious.

I could have drawn this lesson on rational therapeutics from another source, a source, I think, even of more profound interest. It has been said, and said plentifully, that the dawning interest in ailments of the aging is the result of social pressure. Formerly that pressure was exercised, as now in the case of poliomyelitis, to secure protection from bacterial or kindred diseases, because they, often being contagious, were dangerous and required quarantine. Comparable pressure is being exercised now because the ailments incident to older age are incapacitating, long-drawn-out and tend to be costly—indeed very costly. The study of mortality statistics created awareness of this situation; deaths from certain causes were increasing. In the course of a few years a general conception of what this meant has begun to be clear—or clearer. Little still is known. The study of aging began then in a more serious fashion.

The problem what and how to study this period in human life is not, in some respects, unlike that in cancer. What causes aging? Is it necessary or is it preventable? If preventable, does it result from subtle injuries inflicted in the course of ordinary living—injuries to be traced to infection or to diet or to other environmental moments? Where is essential evidence to be sought of the basic mechanism? In changes in the arteries or in some other tissue or organ? Is its cause a substance secreted within the organism—a prime mover, initiating a master reaction—begun not by design, though that is not an unusual conception, but because of its fortuitous and unforeseeable nature? If aging is the result of any of these agents, obviously means to bring the business to a standstill can conceivably be found. But if it should turn out that it is none of these or none comparable to them, but that aging is on the contrary universal, it will be necessary to turn to the conception that aging takes place in the nature of things, is in fact implicit in nature, that somehow it is incidental to living, an expression of the togetherness of the organism, not a follow the leader, or master mechanism; that the disabilities and ailments to which aging gives rise call for alleviation of disability and suffering, different—

or perhaps not different—from those ailments for which relief is sought on the assumption of the preventability of the process.

From the point of view of research, the meaning of all of this is clear. The resources of intelligence are wanted badly—students of natural history, statisticians, morphologists, chemists of several sorts, physiologists, physicians. There may be short cuts to discoveries in this category of disability, but the history of science does not encourage the expectation that one is to be found. It is more likely that in order to learn what to do, it is necessary first to search out the forces that are at work, and the precise forms they assume. Attempts to anticipate solutions by short cuts have too often been futile. It is obvious that not enough is known to make a solution possible. Nor is it now believed that genius can advance far beyond current knowledge. Newton, for example, is unthinkable as a contemporary of Aristotle. Failure in scientific research is often the natural answer to premature adventure. The frequency of simultaneous discoveries is evidence for the correctness of this view. Pressing on the door of the unknown is nowadays constantly taking place. But we do not know beforehand who will force an entrance. We believe, therefore, in freedom of research —one of the academic freedoms which ought, accordingly, sedu-ously to be preserved. Whether a research can be made to pay is a matter of judgment. Who has this judgment? Experience counts of course, though the inexperienced, like Parsifal, often see the light. But Aristotle, Harvey, Young, Helmholtz, Pasteur, Hering, Ludwig, Gaskell, Darwin, to name only biologists were not inexperienced. Since chance enters the calculation, there is little room for dogma.

The clinic, that is to say the hospital, has been an integral part in the scheme for providing for the care and study of patients and their ailments. The fact that clinics offer the opportunity of ob-serving the manifestations exhibited by patients and of comparing them has facilitated greatly, as Shryock has pointed out, the de-scription and classification of diseases. To be able to do this is, as is now known, indispensable in the development of scientific knowledge. When the stage of analyzing the appearances of diseases is reached, the equipment possible to clinics is essential. Equipment includes, for example, laboratories for chemical analyses, for the study of the physiological and physical aspects of diseases, for bacteriology, serology, immunity, hematology. In the past one hundred years, but more especially in the past thirty, such opportunities have actually been provided on a fair scale. It has become possible for physicians to study whatever phase of a disease seems important. Naturally clinics do not neglect the management of patients. On the contrary. They exist for the sole purpose of encouraging better and proper treatment, as adequate as contemporary knowledge permits. It is illuminating to observe how quickly the general public has learned to find its way to university clinics in the belief that the latest information on the cure of diseases is to be found there, where the search for their causes and nature is actively going on. The fear, once entertained, that patients dread examinations by students and are unwilling to subject themselves to novel procedures even though undertaken with proper precautions has been found not to exist or to have been much exaggerated. How to carry on clinical research is one of the lessons which has been learned.

Now, what can be successfully undertaken in the way of research in clinics depends on several factors. It is obvious that the subjects for research are diseases which the patients admitted to a clinic present—these being presumably representative of the forms of illness present in a community. Certain illnesses can be profitably studied—others not. It would for example have been futile for Borelli or for von Helmont in the 17th and 18th Centuries to study infectious diseases. Underlying and contributory knowledge was not yet available.

In the choice of subjects, what I have been calling the level of organization counts—and counts heavily. A distinguished biologist of the past generation spoke often to his friends of the uselessness of investigating diseases until more was known about the behavior of cells, the ultimate proximate constituents composing animals and plants. In certain directions his view was undoubtedly sound. But sera, like those used successfully in treating certain pneumonias or in diphtheria; or a drug like quinidine; or bacteria as causes of diseases; or fibrillation of the auricles as underlying a striking disorder of the heart beat—all these can be, have been, and are being studied to the great benefit of man without carrying on the investigation at a level of organization much below that on which the whole organism as a going concern carries on. It goes without saying that every analysis reduces an organism to a level simpler than that which is being analyzed. That is the condition of analysis. But how far below? I have been saying, not very far, because relevant knowledge is usually not available on a level too far below that at which the phenomenon, that is the object of inquiry, exists. In analyzing morbid processes, the opportunity should be chosen to carry on an investigation at that level precisely, where an experienced or an especially gifted person decides an investigation may be profitable.

Objection is raised on occasion to affording opportunity for thoroughgoing research in clinics, the point being that that opportunity should be sought elsewhere either because elsewhere the cost, financially, may be less; or because the inclusion elsewhere of that research may be more appropriate; or because historically there is value in retaining that study at the locus of its origin. But this is a workaday world; it is difficult to get things done anywhere; men carry on, each his own business and do that with difficulty and against odds. Answers are sought because they are needed. Pathological anatomists, for example, are often in despair because of the lacunae, of great importance to them, left by anatomists. The situation is exactly similar when clinicians require information not supplied by physiologists. But even if anatomists and physiologists have developed a subject, there can be no obligation upon them to go on with it. They may not be aware of the need of a next step. To those to whom taking it is necessary, it is scant comfort to know where preliminary investigations were or should be carried on, if they are no longer being housed there. The fructification of ideas cannot be shackled to a building or even to a locality. But even if the study of a subject is duplicated, the loss is usually not great. Identity in result is rare, mutual criticism is profitable, slight differences in procedure are desirable. There must of course be some sort of common sense on what is investigated in clinics; no one now (1946) would have regarded it as sensible to establish a laboratory for the study of electrons. But such researches as on the metabolism of bacteria, on nomograms describing acid-base and other equilibria, the location and behavior of salts and water, the mechanism of respiratory ferments or of muscular contraction and a host of others is appropriate. To afford hospitality in clinics for such studies seems wholly reasonable. So will domiciling other activities, when the principles involved are scrutinized and understood, such as describing long-drawn-out diseases and senescent states, especially when the interest in them is peculiar to the clinic, and the emphasis necessarily different from that given to them anywhere else.

The decisive question finally arises as to whether men exist in clinics willing to devote themselves to investigations at fundamental levels. Though enterprises at such levels are relatively new, it appears already that little or no difficulty is being experienced. If there is difficulty it exists perhaps in the temptation to draw to too practical purposes, the labors of those who should be, and wish to be, studying at simpler because more manageable levels where the methods of science can be employed. But if so-called fundamental researches are fostered, the possibility exists of guiding them within pragmatic limits and of acquainting clinicians with the value of such enterprises. Against the cost, if the cost is high, must be balanced the motives, the interest in, the concern for the subject. It seems too theoretical to expel from clinics what can be done there more profitably than it can be elsewhere, especially when a clinical interest meets with no outside echo. There are things more expensive than money.

The discussion on the nature of the medical clinic has not, I believe, these many years past, given due significance to these more general aspects of its life. Primary attention has been focused on practice and on teaching because they seemed to be more urgent. These three, teaching, practice and research can, of course, be conducted as co-ordinate functions. The devotion to practice and to teaching must in no sense be whittled away. But it will not be, if the experience of recent years is a guide. What is wanted is a realization that in university clinics, all scholars need not be cut according to the same pattern. Traditionally the roles of teacher and practitioner have been emphasized—perhaps overemphasized. But a clinic affords opportunity for the display of diverse talents; there can be doubt no longer that men of diverse talents can find happiness and opportunity there. To arrive at the precise specifications should not, within this framework, be too difficult. If the conviction begins to prevail that these various functions should find their home there, their adjustment and accommodation may safely be left to the slow, but, one would hope, not too slow, operations of time.

The crucial point is that, to succeed, research in medicine must be regarded a serious undertaking. For whatever reasons, the issues are now regarded as sufficiently urgent by the general public, so that government is devoting increasing attention to the health of the community. To take this problem seriously means that scholars in medicine must be permitted to be serious, as are those in other callings. Education for research must of course be adequate. Free and suitable opportunities for research must exist. And the rewards for service must be ample. Candid, frequent and free criticism must be cultivated. In a technological sense this has been sharp. Experimental nonsense is not lightly tolerated. From a more general point of view—that dealing with the purposes and direction of research, criticism seems to be less well informed. Criticism of a kind can be found in presidental addresses, but the vigor, insight and fearlessness displayed is perhaps not sufficiently incisive. To choosing the direction of investigation, on cultivating precise and incisive forms of debate, more energy can conceivably be devoted than has been customary.

This is what I understand the meaning of medical research to be. The study of diseases has been separated in a category somewhat different from that of the other sciences. That has been due in part to the nature of its subject matter being, in a limited sense, less enduring than that taken for analysis in the other sciences. It has been due in part also to the lateness with which analytical methods have been employed in the study of diseases. The use of them is in full swing now but, being new, the education of men eager to employ them has not been adequately conceived to this end. For this reason also, a critical approach to the analysis of diseases has not yet fully evolved.

Of the objects of human interest, diseases are far from the least. The need for getting on with the understanding of many widespread maladies is urgent. These are very varied, and require for their elucidation professional insight and equipment of a high order. The problems are becoming not less, but more intricate, the more the methods of empiricism change from crude to less crude. The meaning of medical research is to understand the mechanisms at play in diseases and to be concerned with their alleviation and cure.

First published in *Bulletin of the New York Academy of Medicine* (Volume 14, May, 1938).

Changes in Public Attitudes Toward Medicine: Historical Aspects

THE TASK which I have undertaken, of presenting this particular aspect of the history of medical practice, is more difficult than I anticipated. The history is long—as long as there is any writing at all. It is varied, going through all the conceptual relations known to the history of medicine. The search for the succession of practices leads first, all about the basin of the Eastern Mediterranean and later, about the North Atlantic litoral. This history is not the history of medicine only—of medicines and of a knowledge of diseases, but directs attention to the fundamental beliefs of successive generations of men concerning their place in nature, their relation to deity and destiny, as well as to their conception of the nature of diseases. It seems not to be true that, having caught hold of one end of a thread, this can be traced through concentric circles of a labyrinth until the center is reached. There appears to be no such single, continuous thread. There appear to be, even in the limited portion of Mediterranean and Atlantic geography not one thread, but several. The thread has been broken—once when the high Egyptian culture of the Ebers papyrus (1560 B.C.) fell into retrogression; again when Greco-Roman medicine lost its sense of objective reality to give place to medieval supernaturalism; and again wherever empiricism gave way to anti-intellectualism. For, if diseases are part of the natural order, what is meant by any society oriented naturalistically toward natural phenomena, is an attempt at understanding diseases, as if they were part of that natural order. Diseases in this sense, are natural phenomena and are analyzable, therefore, as are other natural phenomena. Reason and the external physical world must constantly be at grips with each other. The effort must constantly be made to discover whether in the light of reason, the natural system works. Actually, so far as therapeutics goes, mankind waited until late in the 17th Century to discover, in the application of a remedial agent, a test of "does it work," when estimated by a statistical method. Therapeutics is not, of course, the only one of the concerns of medical critics but it is, as we shall see, dominant so far as the public attitude to medical practice is concerned. And rightly. For the public need care less about what practitioners think than whether what they think, works well for them.

But beside the level of general culture of a society and the popular conceptions current of the nature of diseases, an insight into the total situation can be gained and from this an understanding of the form of education offered to persons intending to engage in the practice of medicine. I say "total situation" meaning to imply that a society not hard-headed in one or several directions, is unlikely to be so in others. Whatever the central theme of any society, the expectation is that it will push vigorously its conceptions to make the complexion of its public life of a piece. That would be true of the Greeks in the 5th Century or the Romans in the 2nd Century, or medieval Europe in the 13th Century, or modern Europe in the mid-19th Century. It is not without surprise, in western Europe, in a major movement extending 1000 years between the flowering of Greek hard-headedness and the Renaissance, that life was oriented to considerations of spiritual salvation, to salvation of the soul, divorced predominantly from the practical concerns of this planet. At other times the search has lain in regions in which men sought their good in that interaction between reason and the physical world to which I have referred.

There is a relation between discovery and the stimulation of the public imagination which discovery precipitates. When so much is going on that seems to do good to the public, information of the trend being circulated in the public press, the desire grows to participate in the new development. But even more, every physician learns of patients, and there are many, who prefer the buoyancy of faith, to the ministrations, no matter how "scientific," of rational physicians. Such patients prefer faith healers, Christian

Scientists, anyone indeed who aids them as persons, sensitive and passionate, to physicians who watch but can confessedly do nothing, or little. When the choice occurs between psychological help and mechanistic impotence, decision on the part of patients is not difficult. Naturally the division of the whole sea of maladies into these two possibilities is becoming less unequal: The hope is that mechanism, even a knowledge of psychological mechanism, will become ever greater. The shift actually is taking place. The common man is beginning to believe that the form of medicine practiced by scientifically trained physicians has value for him.

How the public attitude toward medicine is changing requires to be defined. Because men are afflicted before birth, in youth, and finally and perhaps most grievously in old age, an attitude toward ailment is inescapable. Historians of medicine usually begin their account of the evolution of medicine by speculating on what assumptions were made before record keeping was practiced. It is assumed, no doubt correctly, that men sought causes for the occurrence of their ailments. And in seeking causes, they sought also remedies. The scene was set for healers of some—as we shall see, of several—sorts. In short, irrespective of theories, men began to take cognizance of the existence of affliction by disease and organized means to defend themselves against their injuries.

The means they employed lie too far back in history to make it at all clear how the attempt at defense began. Surviving records do not suggest that a single system had been developed—not concerning mechanisms of affliction, not concerning the techniques of remedy, not concerning the education of personnel nor its social and professional status. All these came much later. Diseases, therapeutics, healers, belong to no intellectual or scientific scheme that can be identified as organized. The functions of healers depended no doubt on the varieties of ailment. There must have been many just as there are now. And there is evidence that there were specialists—for infections, for the removal of stones, for the setting of bones. Care must have been taken of pregnant women and certainly of parturition. And care must have been taken of the insane or the partially insane. Directly the notion prevailed that against an ailment there existed a remedy, the way must have lain open to inquire would the remedy work, was a remedy needed, how long would healing take? Prognosis in short was born. To this end, signs, portents, symptoms, experience must have counted. That some did, is known from available, relevant evidence.

Therapy conceivably depends on causes. If it does to some extent now, it did not always. If diseases were punishment by the gods for sin and consisted of the invasion of the body by deities or demons or spirits, these were the things to be got rid of, to be exorcised. Somebody had to attend to the exorcism—the patient and someone else, one or both. The conception called for non-mechanistic interference and the organization of a non-rational therapeutic system. Some forms of ailment could be taken care of in this fashion—not stones or broken bones or delivery. The Ebers papyrus mentions physicians, priests, and exorcists. There should be no astonishment that these healers existed side by side. They do, even in our day.

The Greeks seem to have discovered that diseases were natural processes—something dependent on physiology. It was Professor Whitehead who said something to the effect that there is no first-rate idea in the modern world but had its origin in ancient Greece. This idea is one of them. But in Greece as in Babylonia and in Egypt, types of healers ran along side by side.

Irrespective of causes, or if one but knew, in direct relation to certain causes, patients resorted to special types of persons and to special kinds of establishments. Patients with stones and fractures would probably not flock to temples, oracles, or spas. But patients possessed, a word which obviously suggests demoniac or animistic conceptions, would—and so would people with forms of disease that failed to yield to simple local remedies. So would those whose ailments were regarded as visitations of gods, saints, or demons. They would be suffering from diseases regarded as, in some way, connected with sin, retribution, and religion. If the cause were sin or transgression, atonement or appeasement should be sought and perhaps granted, according to the religious belief. The great healers would be those who exercised greatest powers in a religious hierarchy—Asklepios or Christ or the Saints.

It is not necessary to go further into the ramifications implicit in this state. What is essential is to recognize that there was appropriateness in what patients did—that the relief which they sought was sensible for the kind of illness which was manifest.

Men met the challenge of diseases in different ways, depending on the state of their intellectual sophistication. Without an inductive system no matter how primitive, an accurate analysis of the relation of cause and effect was not possible. Since cures depend on causes and since the causes of diseases, especially certain diseases, were believed to depend on deity or more especially on deities, each concerned with a special form of disease, it is not remarkable that the care of diseased persons was associated closely with the practice of religion and rested in the hands of priests. Priests arrogated this function to themselves. What the priests knew they kept to themselves; they formed a cult. They did, in Greece. There have been times even in the Christian era when Church and the clergy fought lay practitioners for attempting to assume this burden.

It is impossible to describe fully the changing conditions of practice in successive periods during the 2500 years past. It is enough to record briefly:

1. The Egyptian and Greek situation
2. The condition in the Middle Ages
3. The way of things in the modern world

Even without details, the broad outlines emerge clearly. In the origin of institutions, whether in Mesopotamia, Egypt, Crete and Greece, mythological persons assume dramatic roles. Gods and goddesses, men and women, act out their parts on a mythological stage. When the historical scene opens, they have accomplished their ends. In the Trojan war, Homer introduces physicians and surgeons who perform their parts. They respond to the needs of war, as if a tradition of learning and of practice were already well established. Certain of the ways of healing had been blocked out—in surgery, the care of fractures, dislocations and stone; in medicine, the use of drugs, inunctions, purgations. This is lay, not priestly, medicine. Similar developments existed also in Egypt

Both in Egypt and in Greece there are records—in Egypt especially the Smith and Ebers papyri make clear what diseases were recognized, what remedies were available. In Greece there is a succession of information, in Homer, in the fragments of inscriptions found in the ruins of the temples and the schools, in the Hippocratic writings. Later, there are the writings of Celsus, Oribasius, Paulus Aegineta. Alongside temple medicine, rational, empirical medicine developed. That is the medicine later recognized as Hippocratic. The practitioners were craftsmen and seem to have been taught *mutatis mutandis* much as physicians are taught now—they observed, they classified, they reconstructed the natural history of diseases. They made efforts at developing useful drugs.

Lay medicine seems to have been well established on the Greek mainland. There were full time physicians employed by larger communities who received public, but who besides were permitted to charge private, fees. In smaller towns physicians picked up what practice they could selling their knowledge as other vendors sold their commodities. Since there was no method of licensing physicians, whoever wished to engage in practice and to treat patients for fees could do so. These men were professionals who, as Sigerist has pointed out, had as one of their chief recommendations the reputation for success which they had acquired. Reputation was capital. All of this seems, but is not certain, to have antedated the establishment of religious medicine. How religious medicine arose is obscure. Gods and goddesses overlooked the care of patients suffering from different classes of diseases. For them, in selected regions, shrines were built in appropriate places, selected with regard to the advantages of climate and of beauty of location. Sometimes there were springs of mineral waters. When such shrines became popular, their wealth increased until great establishments were built, as at Epidauros which began to flourish before the 5th Century. In the course of time there was built a fine temple to Asklepios, a theater, gymnasia, stadia and a hippodrome. There were dormitories for patients, just as at Saratoga, or Baden Baden or Bath or Vichy. Pausanias described his visit to Epidauros in the 2nd Century A.D. This spa has a continuous history accord-

ingly for a period not less than 600 years, drawing patients fro॑
far and wide. Since little is known affirmatively of the beginning॑
either of lay or of temple medicine in Greece, there is no nee॑
now to date one in terms of the other. What is reasonably ce॑
tain is, that lay medicine was practiced alongside temple medicin॑

It seems possible to distinguish between what the priests did an॑
what the physicians. Physicians took care of the common, acu॑
ailments and injuries; the priests, of patients suffering fro॑
chronic diseases which were treated at temple establishments wit॑
exercises, baths and inunctions. More important though, one ma॑
guess, were neuroses, psychoses, obscure ailments like anemias an॑
sterility in men, but especially in women. The priests, one ma॑
be certain, wrapped about what they did in mystery, for whic॑
rituals existed of various degrees of elaborateness. Purification ॑
mind, but especially of the body, played its role. Dreams were inte॑
preted, hypnotic states were induced. The healing dream playe॑
obviously an important part in cures. When Pausanias visite॑
Epidauros, he was shown votive tablets recording the names ॑
patients and the diseases of which they were cured, the metho॑
of treatment that was used. The inscriptions, in order to mak॑
sense, require skill in interpretation; in their inscribed form the॑
appear, sometimes, utterly incomprehensible. On the whole cur॑
in the temples take on a miraculous complexion, as in the far॑
tastic story of Aristagora of Troixenes.

For the training of priests there were undoubtedly temp॑
schools in which the mysteries were handed on, generation afte॑
generation, as is the custom in esoteric cults.

Parallel with the temple spas and the temple schools were th॑
lay schools of Cyrene, Rhodes, Cnidos and Cos. That Cos wa॑
not a temple school, is suggested by the fact that in the who॑
Hippocratic Corpus, there is no mention of a miraculous cur॑
What the temper and the nature of instruction in lay schools wa॑
appears from Hippocratic writings. Observations, descriptions, in॑
ference, the method of experiment, a form of rude statistics, under॑
lay their practice. Out of this grew theories of physiology—crise॑
humors, phlegms. It was sound system, directly comparable t॑
what, in natural history, Aristotle was doing in the 4th Century॑

What went on in the Greek lay schools remained the basis of thought until the Renaissance.

What the Greek philosophic schools, what Alexandria, and Roman medicine added, were some adventures in anatomy and in physiology with which the names of Herophilus and of Erasistratus (ca. 310-250 B.C.), of Galen and other Greco-Roman physicians, are prominently connected. Actually it is not clear that after the Greek Foundations there is significant development in the comprehension of diseases such as would influence what patients could expect in the way of cures, until the time of the Renaissance. In Rome there was a time, in the empire, when the social position of physicians seems to have been not unsatisfactory; Julius Caesar made them citizens in 46 B.C.; medical schools were founded in Pergamum, Marseilles, Lyon, Saragossa, Antioch. But whatever the power of rational thought, it had neither the strength nor the originality to maintain the spark of reason against increasing popular reliance on on-rushing competitors from the East which brought into Rome beliefs and cults as irrational as was the temple medicine in Greece. It was again a situation in which mystical medicine, temple medicine, flourished side by side with the medicine of the rational schools.

With the coming of the Christian era, those forces were at work which sapped the strength of the social and intellectual life of the empire. Wars, pestilence, poverty, the disinherited, the rising masses of the underprivileged, the hard and lower standards of living, epidemics, all these combined to render men careless of what had been the opportunities and the rewards of the rich and powerful in the preceding centuries. The cultivation of health so dear to the Greeks, the cultivation of luxurious living, apparently so indispensable to the privileged Romans, were no longer ways of life to be envied. For common men, theirs was not the way along which hope was to be found. New motives became apparent. Old motives received new emphasis. Insistence on interdependence is one. Professor Sigerist regards the brotherhood motive in primitive Christianity as determining—in the sense that men are responsible for one another, in sickness and in health, that Christians form a vast family, the members of which assume responsibility for each other. This motive accounts for the fact that communities as wholes, have throughout this era charged themselves in theory at least, with the public care of the unfortunate. This motive accounts for the establishment and maintenance of hospitals and other institutions for the care of the sick. There can be little doubt that the recognition of communal responsibility constitutes a turning point in the attitude of the public.

But there is another aspect of the matter, for which the acceptance of Christianity by the Mediterranean world is also responsible. The general social and economic conditions which were prevalent in the centuries before and after the beginning of this era, made it desirable to pin the hopes of the vast majority of people on something other than the possibility of material well being. That there was no comfort in this world, that so far as its goods went, most men were underprivileged, turned attention away from that chance of betterment, which depended on goods and things. They were ready to be taught to look for religious equivalents of salvation—salvation for the spirit instead of the gratification of the flesh. The new way, which despised the body but sought instead salvation for the soul, found in the Roman proletariat a congenial soil. The world of rational arrangements, the world of rational thinking, the world of rational medicine, was at an end. Privilege meant advantage of one man over another, because of wealth or position. What could be bought was for the advantage of the body. In the new dispensation, privilege was cast out and in its place came a new feeling for man, for his intrinsic worth. A theory was adopted which made men brothers, which made them mutually dependent, which made salvation a business of the soul, and neglect of the body, a virtue. These new values destroyed the values of the ancient world. For Christian society, wealth and the advantages of wealth disappeared. For the new poor, lay physicians and lay practice had accordingly no meaning. The Greek and Roman systems for the support of medical practice disappeared. Since the care of illness could no longer be a private concern, it became a communal enterprise.

In this content, there could be no other outcome than the sub-

stitution of irrationality for rationality—and to make of that substitution, a thorough-going reconstruction of the tenets which
applied to the whole of social organization. This substitution went
so far that in the 2nd Century A.D., Christian students of Galen
were excommunicated for devoting their time to the study of
pagan medicine. Later, in the 12th Century, when the medieval
church was in the heyday of its power, the anti-intellectual tendency was strong enough to forbid Benedictine friars from cultivating the study of medicine—the Benedictines especially having held
learning in some sort of esteem. The practice of the Benedictines
did in fact keep alive something of the rational Greek tradition.
There is much evidence that, instead of having disappeared completely, as is so often assumed, that strain which began to develop
again powerfully in the 14th and 15th Centuries, runs as a faint
trickle through medieval thought. Faint, because its significance
was scarcely made much of. For modern scholars the copying of
manuscripts has made endless trouble through the corrupt copying
of the ancient texts by monks who undertook this labor, or to
whom it was assigned, not for the love of learning, but as punishment in the expiation of sin. The ancient literature was, nevertheless, in this fashion, kept alive. It had its influence.

The motives underlying the care of the sick in the medieval
church may have been different from those which activated priests
in Egyptian temple medicine. The motive of charity, later exemplified by St. Francis, may have been enough. The fact seems to be
that no other group of individuals was trained or had the leisure
to undertake this service. Clerics did in fact take it on. In time
there came to be established monastic medicine. Throughout the
early Middle Ages, religious orders served these functions—the
Templars, the Knights of St. John, and later, more especially,
the Benedictines. At the zenith of their concern with sickness they
taught at widely separated stations—at Montecassino, at Oxford,
at Cambridge, at Tours, at Fulda and at St. Gall.

The care of the sick, obviously, was a time-consuming business.
There came to be criticism of this activity on two counts; the
brothers devoted too much of their time away from the monas-
teries; they were developing a degree of rationality, of scholar-

ship, at variance with the best interests of the ecclesiastical establishment.

But before the end, long before the end of this movement, seed was sown which, when it began properly to flourish, flowered into a plant of such strength and vigor, that it still nourishes the current system. The Benedictines from Montecassino in the 7th Century founded a hospital, at the salubrious site of Salerno. There the sick began to congregate. Later, in the 10th Century, the school of Salerno was founded. Later still Frederick II promulgated rules for general and special education which may still be regarded with admiration and may still serve as guides to conduct. Later still, faculties of medicine, imitative of the school of Salerno began to flourish everywhere in Western Europe.

In a sense what went on at the school of Salerno is shrouded in mystery. In another, enough is known so that it is possible for the learned to be learned about it. Actually Salerno serves well as a symbol. It was a focal point for the meeting of the persons and ideas beginning again to be abroad. There was a mixture of irrational and rational, but more especially a breaking through of the rational. Egyptians, Constantinus Africanus, Jews, Saracens, Northern Europeans, foregathered—Germans, it was the day of the Hohenstaufens, and Italians. Greek, Hebrew and Arabic were understood. In Sicily, closely adjoining, the three languages are said to have been used simultaneously like their successor languages in New York. And here also for the first time in the Christian learned world, women began to play a role. It makes no difference whether Trotula existed—that there should be debate about the possibility of her activity, is enough to establish the fact that the tight structure of the social web was loosening.

And out of all this came a book, in many versions, in many languages in countless editions (500 according to L. Choulant). The *Regimen Sanitatis* attained fame and captured the hygienic imagination of Europe, as had Pliny's natural history, its intellect. Sir John Harington, responsible for the greatest of European revolutions through the invention of the water closet, translated this work (1607). It taught many things—as to the maintenance of health, as to household remedies, as to sensible daily behavior.

Knowledge of this book must have traveled far and wide. It must have been a powerful lever in elevating the minds of people from the bog of ignorance to the upper air of roaming inquiry.

That a book like this should have been produced is indicative merely of the temper of a time. This book was not its only sign. Albertus Magnus, far away at Cologne, wrote his natural history. The mere mention of these names, of Arnald of Villanova, of Mondino, are enough to make clear in what directions the minds of common men were stirring. The exclusive sway of the religions was over; there was room for new things.

In the later Middle Ages, when laymen again were attracted to the profession of medicine, it was again possible to render services for pay. The Church employed many physicians, as did also men in the upper levels of the social hierarchy. The powerful and rich employed physicians for public services, and in the interests of their personal care.

By the end of the 15th Century, a new dispensation was firmly established—there were well-organized schools; there were rules which governed medical practice; there were penalties for illegal practices; for practitioners without licenses. Practice, finally, attempted to tear away from the faculties of the cathedral and university schools and fell increasingly in the hands of the laity.

But the irrational strains, never lost in Greek and Roman temple medicine, continued to flourish under the auspices of the medieval church. Gods became saints. It was the saints that the afflicted appealed to, for protection and relief. It was saints who presided over shrines and spas and baths. Demons and spirits continued to possess the mentally sick, and clerics, witches and sorcerers continued to exorcise them. In many cases as a last resort help was sought in the laying on of hands—miraculous cures were reported, owing even to the royal touch of an anointed king. The appeal of irrational, religious, temple medicine was still powerful. The persons and the auspices and the system were different, but the thing in itself was still the same. The need for help was as imperative as ever, and that help could not be supplied by a rational system when reason had made advances so slight as to offer scant comfort to those in acute suffering.

As the centuries wore on and the Renaissance dawned in the
14th and 15th Centuries, a rearrangement in emphasis among the
various medical strains had taken place. The interests of people
in Western Europe were drawn again toward interest in this
world. The crusades unsettled the crystalline sediment of the
more ancient cultures. Looking outward instead of exclusively
inward, stirred the old crystals into circulation and rendered fluid
whạt had been precipitated. The westward migration of Greek
scholars and the northward migration of their Arabic and Hebrew
colleagues served to disturb the stagnant pools. That this evolution should have taken place is in the nature of things, which,
whether we like it or not, continuously change. The world forced
attention upon itself and began again to be reckoned with. The
scholars, the crusades, the migrations, the needs of religion itself,
chanced merely to have been the instruments of change. Finally,
the Moslems, having shut off Europe both from Eastern Asia by
their impenetrable crescent formed by Transjordania, Egypt and
North Africa, and also from the rest of the faintly remembered
world farther to the East, stimulated the maritime discoveries of
the 15th and 16th Centuries. These processes and adventures together, succeeded in prodding the minds of men to inquiry—
encouraging them inescapably, even if, to many thoughtful persons, reluctantly. The materials for a new revolution were now
forged.

In the history of medicine heroes also have their uses. They
serve as symbols. Philippus Aureolus Theophrastus Bombastus
Paracelsus von Hohenheim (1493-1541) would serve as one even
without his high-sounding name. But his name itself is a clarion.
It is onomatopoetic. It announces a new time; it boasts properly,
as when one is uncertain whether to boast at all. All the ancient
strains of medical thought and practice are focused in him. But he
symbolizes beside enough augury of the time to come. He gives one
the self-confident feeling of spring. He spoke his own language;
people understood him. He had the assurance of one who thought
he knew how to stand alone. Within himself he combined both
rational and irrational motives. Feeling his strength, alive to
events and interests which had been suppressed, he cut a wide

swathe in the world of his day. He doubted, he inquired, he experimented. He taught people to throw away crutches, he breathed faith in himself and in reason. He reminded people that they must look upon the world afresh, that their teachers were ignorant, that they must search themselves. He symbolized the self-reliant dawn —wisely forgetful of the dawn of yesterday. Whatever was outmoded and useless in concept or practice that Paracelsus and his time inherited from the past, they were ready to discard—they were ready for the forward march. Paracelsus is a brave symbol —fit to stand beside Leonardo and Galilei.

One would have thought that after Paracelsus, witches, religious healing, pilgrimages to sacred spas, magic, belief in improbable or impossible miracles would disappear. But they did not disappear nor did therapeutics become a well-thought-out enterprise. Everybody was not impressed with Descartes's *Discourse on Method*— not many even of those who knew of it were influenced by its plain teaching.

But the complexion of things changed gradually nevertheless. The universities planted herb gardens; they tried out the efficacy of their extracts. The barbers became surgeons. Medical people began to observe diseases studiously, to compare them and to assemble like cases. They began to draw inferences from their resemblances in order to describe, to classify, to prognosticate. What the professors learned, the populace soon began to know. They began to travel again in search of cures—not to the holy places, not to the temples, but to the professors themselves, to the university clinics—to Leyden, to Vienna.

After the motives of the Renaissance had been gaining momentum some two or three centuries, when travel became freer and speculation bolder, new considerations entered upon the scene, considerations which originated in the very changes in life and thought and trade that were transforming Europe and which reached their full stride at the end of the 17th Century in England. Populations in western European countries were still small— 19,000,000 in France, 5,500,000 in England and Wales. With increase in the means of production, with the expansion of foreign markets, increase in population became desirable, and the preservation of the existing small populations available became imperative.

The Christian insistence on the mutual interdependence of men survived. Out of this the sense of humaneness became intensified and also the desirability of private and certainly of public philanthropy. The founding of hospitals expanded. But in the 17th and 18th Centuries new motives became dominant. Men, always valuable became more valuable still. This motive, beyond that of brotherly love, compelled inquiry into the conditions of living. How long did men live? Of what did they die? Could one, by being informed of such matters, improve the state of affairs? Now enter upon the scene the names of authentic well-known personages—mathematicians and statisticians—like Sir William Petty and later of the first actuaries, of Johann Peter Frank and of other men interested in the public health.

In the year of the Declaration of Independence, Johann Peter Frank, Court Physician to the Sovereign Bishop of Speyer, is a figure of arresting interest. He addressed a circular "Letter of Invitation to Scholars to Send the Decrees of Rulers and Legislators relating to Medical Polity" to him. This letter runs as follows:

Gentlemen,

That the preservation of the health of peoples and states and the multitude of regulations necessary for this purpose are of great importance will certainly not be doubted when it is realized that the inseparable accompaniment of true happiness, namely bodily health, while it runs many a risk of being neglected, also contributes largely to the increase of the common weal.

Rulers, being destined by nature to set an example, have at last recognized the importance of this matter and have therefore been establishing of late in various districts those famous public health boards whose special concern it is to eradicate anything that is injurious to the public well-being and to promote anything that tends to preserve and increase the health of the citizens.

Owing, however, to the wide range of the subject and to the fact that the policy is still much too new to have found general assent, many factors, and those certainly not the least important for improving the public health, have had to be ignored. A closer enquiry will make clear to educated persons the duty of investigating the generally overlooked influence of these neglected factors and of deciding in earnest which are suitable for this or that locality and people.

Frank enumerated roughly 17 different functions which his department of health should serve, but, being wise, he doubted whether he had exhausted the possibilities. He turned again to the Scholars:

To you, therefore, Gentlemen, I address my renewed requests and wishes, that you should deem it worth your while kindly to let me know of anything I seem not to have mentioned to you here which might be useful in elucidating this work devoted to humanity, especially any regulations relating to Medical Polity that you know from your experience have been applied with success or are to be applied either here or elsewhere. Please confer with me on these topics by friendly correspondence and, if there should come into your hands any writings worth consulting, lend them with the assurance that I will in each case gratefully and faithfully refund any expenses and, as far as possible, lest I should become a nuisance to any of my patrons, I will conscientiously observe any further conditions that may be imposed.

Enumeration is not a new method to be applied to affairs of State. But it is not an old method either. Recently the centenary of the publication of Quetelet's epoch-making *Social Physics* was celebrated. The importance which this publication has attained, in view of many scholars, becomes manifest when it is pointed out that the copy of this book which was presented by Quetelet to Florence Nightingale has been singled out to be placed side by side, in the Galton Laboratory at University College, with the copy of the *Origin of Species* that Darwin presented to Francis Galton and with the copy of his Belfast address which Tyndall gave to Herbert Spencer. Indeed, the conception that *Social Physics* or, as we should say now, the statistical treatment of social affairs, can yield important insights goes back not even so far as the reign of Queen Elizabeth. That the conception is still young emerges from the fact that this approach to understanding the structure of society and its social needs has won, and still is winning, its way slowly and painfully in important departments of communal life. And nowhere is advance more painful than in the effort to appraise the relative significance of diseases. Captain John Graunt's *Natural and Political Observations upon the Bills of Mortality* appeared in 1662. The first duly licensed edition of Sir William Petty's *Political Arithmetick* written in 1676-77 was published in 1690. And Edmund Halley's "An estimate of the degrees of the mortality of mankind drawn from curious tables of the births and funerals at the city of Breslaw, with an attempt to ascertain the price of annuities upon lives" appeared in 169⅔. How many persons remember that originally "statistics" meant a "description of States," though it has now become a dark science, devoted to what is called a "systematic compilation of instances for the inference of general truths." But though there has been a change in definition of the word "statistics," what has occurred, as Sarton points out, is merely a shift in meaning. Enumeration of occurrences is still, indeed it is becoming, an ever more indispensable method for guiding the affairs of citizens in the hands of competent administrators. It is a mark of her genius that "for Florence Nightingale, Quetelet was the hero as scientist." Between Graunt and Petty and Halley, and ourselves came the valiant Johann Peter Frank. He counted as important, number 16 among the 17 enterprises of his department of health, "the question of the classification of diseases under quite simple heads and the faithful recording of the cause of death in each case. In this way (as he thought) the nature of endemic diseases, i.e., those peculiar to a single region, will at length become clearer and, when the figures are compared with a more accurate computation of the annual number of births, the death rate will be apparent."

This matter of the public health, from then onward, has received greater and ever greater attention. If the problems that required solution were, at first, the problems centering in the prevalence of infectious diseases, that was owing to the great number of young persons affected and to their devastating destructiveness. When, after the successful exploitations that followed an understanding of the influence of bacteria on the occurrence of infectious diseases, the number of such cases diminished enormously, officers and investigators charged with the care of the public health began to turn their attention to other forms of affliction which, after the conquest of the communicable diseases, demanded urgent attention. These are the so-called chronic diseases to be found both among young and old and the disabilities incident to old age.

But these are matters of now.

The great turnover came in the 16th Century with the rise of liberalism. Men fought free of control by all dominant organizations when the method of life since called *laissez faire* was developed. The medical faculties which had grown up under the protection of the Church attempted to retain control through the regulation of medical practice. The errors which they made after the dawn of the new empirical medicine fostered organizations like academies, and other learned societies, to carry on medical studies and medical organization outside the faculties. The struggle in Paris to gain recognition of the discovery that the blood circulates, suggests in a concrete way the kind of battle which the medical faculties carried on with current unorthodox research. The Church in this instance, as in others, fought a losing, rear-guard action. The powers of rationalism were conquering. Novelty is like Pandora's box; when the lid opens unanticipated things fly out. If it was impossible any longer to restrain the curiosity of men, the consequences are not always satisfactory and could not, as one looks back, have resulted otherwise than is now apparent. If men were free they could indulge their impulses; if they indulged their impulses, competition arose; if competition arose there arose iniquity; if there arose iniquity, society defended itself by regulation. And a further consequence of the effort on the part of society to secure what it wishes and needs, is making in our day for re-orientation and new alignments in the technique of the practice of medicine.

All of this was taking place in the early years of the industrial revolution. In its wake, came overcrowding in towns and cities, wretched housing and general insanitary conditions for great masses of workers and of the poor. Poverty, intemperance, industrial diseases became rampant. This situation challenged the indifference of governments. Humanitarians like Robert Owen and Edwin Chadwick, took active parts in attempting to relieve these conditions. The workers themselves fought for better working conditions through unions of their own. Their own alertness, under vigorous leadership like that of Francis Place, went far toward accelerating the pace at which reforms and new services were instituted. This movement became cumulative through the Century until after the turn of the 20th when the government in Great Britain, under the guidance of Mr. Lloyd George, instituted sweeping reforms in the National Insurance Act, whereby authority was granted to assign money, collected by taxation, specifically for public medical purposes. With this money, need for research and for the administration of the public health was met at least in part. With the institution of an arrangement, as suitable as possible, that provided for the paneling of physicians a great forward step was taken. At length the public has become conscious of its democratic right to treatment for its ailments. A new chapter has been opened which has assured men, through being cared for, of a greater measure of enjoyment which is legitimately theirs. When governments charged themselves finally with the hygienic regulation of those industries, occupation in which was attended by danger to the health of working men, a scheme for the full care of the public was in sight.

It is unnecessary to trace this development of public concern for the health and the diseases of individuals further, in different countries, nor according to special means, whether in general hospitals, in lying-in hospitals, in protection against contagious diseases to which the whole public is exposed, nor in the elaborate insurance schemes to aid the middle classes and the poor in securing adequate medical care. The intention here is to do no more than to outline the direction of advance and the action which has been taken. That the people themselves are now aroused is made manifest through their willingness, in the democracies, to permit themselves to be taxed for these purposes.

Side by side with the development of interest by the State in the general public health and specifically in industrial hygiene there evolved another motive, the motive that is expressed in the Christian democratic regard for the value of individual men. If men had value, they had it to better purpose if they could function completely, sound minds in sound bodies. It would be natural to find a basis for such doctrines in the literature of democracy, in John Locke and in J. J. Rousseau.

What emerges from these reflections are generalizations, rough approximations no doubt, very different from what I should have written down had I not been given an opportunity of studying this subject in an orderly fashion. What I found at the outset, when I started arranging my mind in order to write, was that the attitude of populations changed toward things medical. A more careful perspective suggests that this has not been the case. Years in the calendar have not been separated in compartments by horizontal boundaries. That may have occurred at the beginning of those centuries during which the Roman Church set the intellectual and religious pace. The attitude of the peoples has always been dictated by the same motive—the need for help. It has been their attitude, the attitude of the whole of a society, which has decided what small or great shifts from one form of relief to another the state of knowledge and of feeling necessitated. What has not been understood, or perhaps it would be more nearly correct to say, what I have not understood, is that there have always been two strains in what roughly, very roughly, we call medicine. "Always" is itself a rough word. There has always been temple medicine—there has always been rational medicine. They have always existed side by side; they exist side by side now. The philosophy, the general beliefs of a society, dominates its behavior, literally forcing its major emphasis. A mystical, transcendental philosophy necessitates the view that relief is to be gained by irrational practices; a naturalistic philosophy, that rational practice is the only possible adventure. This separation in emphasis is general and distinguishes whole eras. But whatever the intellectual, the philosophical climate, the two strains have persisted. There are three questions:

What in the way of belief shifts?
What diseases are involved?
How do the answers to these questions influence public behavior?

So much having become understood, it became clear also that there are times when temple medicine makes a more prominent appeal, times when rational medicine does, and that whichever is the case depends on the general state of contemporary culture. Where naturalists are in the ascendant, rational medicine will be. So far as diseases go, there is a clear and sharp division among categories. The less understood, the demoniac, the possessed, the mystical, sterility, impregnation, gestation, neurosis, insanity, all these complaints in the category of the inexplicable, of the mysterious, of the God-inflicted—these fall to the priests, the medicine men, the temple healers. Fevers, stones, fractures, dislocations —these fall to rational practitioners, to lay physicians. With advance in learning and the accumulation of critical experience, the area of rational treatment becomes applicable to more and more situations—resort to temple medicine becomes less and less frequent. The hope of rational medicine is that ultimately, understanding will have acquired such power as to make temple medicine, so uncertain in its success, all but superfluous. Reason will have triumphed. More people have slowly been learning how to distinguish between hope and despair. They do not go to the temple for stone or fractures; they tend, fortunately or unfortunately, not to take the insane or the neurotic to the lay physician.

Temple medicine persists in our time. Nothing is gained by ignoring this. The Emanuel movement, the Christian Science movement, the confessional, all are evidence that it does. It succeeds where reason has not yet had opportunity for thoroughgoing exploration. But that time will soon be upon us. The great contribution of Sigmund Freud consists in the effort to analyze what is going on in the minds of men, of collecting that experience, of attempting cures. There are tests of success, in cases which have been cured. Of these Lourdes, Saint Ann de Beaupré and Christian Science can exhibit many and so earn the gratitude of men. But psychoanalysis and its related efforts at mental healing differ from former, irrational, perhaps comparable attempts by insisting upon the critical accumulation of evidence, upon classifying that evidence, and upon drawing rational deductions from it. In the realm of the mind, this is the first time an effort irrespective of the degree of its success has been made that lifts this dark corner of human suffering into the light where the play of reason becomes possible on the road to better understanding.

Where so much of what goes on in the mind and, to fall in with popular conceits, the soul has seemed so elusive in mechanistic medicine, so withdrawn from the possibility of treatment on rational grounds, these recent attempts in psychological medicine give hope that success is not beyond the power of human intelligence. The strongest of Nature's citadels having been stormed successfully, there is hope that the end is in sight, that a better comprehension of the mechanism of abnormal behavior has been attained.

What is difficult to fathom is insight into how opinion on these subjects, temple and rational medicine, has been moving among the people—how much are they addicted to current temple practices—how much do they rebel at rational arrangements which yield such unsatisfactory results? There are those who do. The evidence is to be found in the sharp critical writings, widely scattered in time, of Aristophanes, of Molière, of George Bernard Shaw. Their remarks are straws in the wind of public opinion. Theirs is evidence that scepticism is ancient, intellectual and behavioristic. But they are destructive critics without hope and without faith in the competence of rational men.

If the present, as we are so often told, is to be understood in terms of experience, to reverse the process is also quite fair and so to inquire, how much of what is going on under our very eyes, how much of the present can be used to illuminate the past. There can be no doubt that to appraise that present is extraordinarily difficult. There are now, without doubt, clear evidences of social pressure at work, to force advance in knowledge of diseases. What else can it mean when great Foundations investigate the state of medical education, suggesting and determining at the same time how this can be improved; when others aid county health boards in attempting to manage their local diseases; when men are stimulated to study classes of diseases anew, of insanity, of the blood vessels, or cancer; when still others are moved to investigate a situation like that among the aged; when private philanthropists turn to supplying clean milk to save infants and children from intestinal infection? These are expressions of the fact that laymen, dissatisfied with the state of affairs, have sought and have found ways of bringing pressure to bear on professionals, urging them on to bring about improvements, too long delayed.

Naturally such social activity must not be divorced from what the reflections of a time suggest and make possible. They are part and parcel of it, no doubt. And yet, being done in the way in which it is, it is not chance, but deliberateness that initiates these performances. Anyone who has occasion to read the incoming mail of any prominent institution for medical research will be struck with how much suggestion, some foolish, is furnished by laymen, deeply concerned with the general defects in knowledge and eager to help in remedying this situation.

Yes, the common man and his lay leaders are aroused and, in our day, care. Associations like the Cancer, the Tuberculosis, the Heart Association are evidence of the same solicitude. The problem is to find the way to advancement, how to lay one's hand on the end of Ariadne's silken thread that leads on to the center and so the heart of the labyrinth.

And now, with this experience, is it possible to push back and to try to illuminate the past? In any sense in which our world can be known, that is possible only to the extent that a record of events is available. Unfortunately that record is meager. There is a difference between overwhelming eagerness to make the most elementary provision to improve one's comfort and that of one's neighbor and the hesitation to say nothing of the pusillanimity of corporate bodies to extend the bounds of knowledge. If occasional Greek cities employed physicians to ease the ailments of their citizens there is little reason to think they were active in maintaining institutions for research. If a record of the performances at Cos or at the Museum at Alexandria has come down to us where, under private initiative or under government, systematic investigations at least of anatomy and physiology and surgery were fostered, it would be difficult or impossible to duplicate such experiences until the close of the Middle Ages, at schools like Salerno, as forerunners of what was thought, tried and accomplished, be-

ginning in the 16th Century in the academies of the Italian city
republics and in their successors in England, France and Germany.

What is striking is the evenness with which a whole front moves
forward. That is part of the wonder—the temple part, if after all
that precedes the temple element is still insistent. The single case
of Pasteur is perhaps a perfect illustration. A record of the movement of his mind among such subjects as crystallography, isomer-
ism, specificity, fermentation and diseases of the vine, of silk-
worms, of sheep, and of men—not episodic, but tightly and
intimately concatenated. To cite his case is perhaps to cite the
best one. But other illustrations leap to mind—Goethe, for example, or in our own time, Sir William Hardy and Sir Ernest
Rutherford. If the point can be made in the cases of single minds,
this but points to what is possible and no doubt the rule in societies
of minds.

That evenness of the front, slight pseudopods perhaps excepted,
has seemed on occasion not to have been illustrated in advancing
knowledge of diseases either by individuals or by social pressure.
It is an interesting point, one about which one's view undergoes
shifts. The central question is, could the date of a discovery have
been advanced? What in the way of preliminary knowledge
should have been available? Was there such knowledge? It takes
much knowing to answer such questions. A slight test is a record
of discoveries and inventions that go into the manufacture of the
internal combustion engines of aeroplanes. What would have been
possible at Kitty Hawk had *every* resource then available been put
freely at the disposal of the brothers Wright? Could the trans-
continental machine have been built? It is an idle question to
which there is an obvious answer.

Another test can be made in the case of so-called simultaneous
discoveries. Lists of these have been compiled. The length of them
is, in point of fact, impressive. What they demonstrate is that at
many points, many men are pressing forward, searching meticulously for, in order to pierce, weak places in Nature's secret
armor. And they do often, at widely separated points, practically
simultaneously.

Take the situation at this moment, in cancer, in arterial hypertension, in Bright's disease—to mention only the most obvious of

the challenges offered by diseases. How is Nature's armor here to be pierced? There has been much systematic labor. But have the specifications been drawn for the correct edifice? Who knows except the genius with insight. Here the prepared mind may not be enough. Perhaps it is too early—perhaps a prepared mind cannot yet have been formed. This is the situation that generates hopelessness—the situation that demands persistence, that understands the slowness of the process, that recognizes that the heart of this artichoke is protected by an unforeseeable number of petals and that these must be stripped one by one. The search often breaks the heart of a scientist and may for a while still, leave the heart of the artichoke well protected and undisclosed. Faith here, and hope are what are necessary.

The point need not be labored further. It may be possible, no doubt it is possible, to push forward harder and faster. But it would be difficult to be certain that there is energy available to this end.

Enough has been said to indicate the argument which this discourse seeks to support. There is no need to categorize the ideas for purposes of action. Action, not enough perhaps, not sufficiently varied, not always adequately imaginative, is nevertheless taking place. What is more important is to tear web from woof to understand better the fabric into which the strands which make for its texture are woven. Two or perhaps three have been found. They have a strange, natural relation to one another. They have, as elements, relations of interdependence governed by the deeper thought of successive periods of belief and speculation; but they remain still independent strands, their strength varying with time. In our day we should be content to see the rational strand grow strong in order to make the irrational wholly dispensable. To turn the two about, rational and irrational, we should take as evidence of the loss of our civilization. This is an assignment of value of what we believe is the mechanism of our salvation. Our successors may, of course, reverse our estimates. The history of our kind is checkered and moves on quicksand.

First published in *Bulletin of the New York Academy of Medicine* (Volume 11, January, 1942).

The Difference Between Art and Science in Their Relation to Nature

IT IS not uncommon to believe that Art and Science lie on opposite slopes of a psychological divide, but it is a belief which does not trouble many persons; it is merely accepted. Whatever the problem, it lies beyond the urgencies of these troublous times. And yet, on both sides of the divide, there is wistful awareness that somehow, something is going on on the other which it would be a pity to miss; on the art side, profound new curiosity about science, from physics to psychology. Artists have experienced it before—Leonardo, the Impressionists and their followers. On the science side, men are bewildered because of the use of forms of expression, in painting especially, which are represented as evidence of what goes on in the mind.

Imaginary conversations have been a source of entertainment from Plutarch to Landor. They provide a way of suggesting contrasts which are usually not obvious. Often, the result is illuminating. That kind of confrontation is what this essay attempts. Familiar views are made to take on unfamiliar shapes under a shadow-casting exploring light. Science and Art have not often been examined in this kind of juxtaposition. Something may be gained from this adventure.

I. INTRODUCTORY

"Art" is a loose term. It includes the "fine arts," sculpture, poetry, painting, and music, but only the most elevated examples in these kinds—not applied art nor the lesser forms of expression.

Science will not be taken to mean applied science, the application of the result of scientific thought or of fundamental scientific discovery to the affairs of the everyday world. That way lies invention. Science is insight. Science is that effort which men keep making to understand this world and the universe and besides the methods used in that undertaking. Science, pure science, is one way of looking at nature—nothing more. No part of the world is omitted—not the infinitely large nor yet the infinitely small. The ways of nature have not failed to challenge the passionate interest of the most inquisitive of men. Success in bringing into some comprehensible scheme the welter of observations, of facts, and of ideas has been the good fortune of those who have been possessed of the most imaginative, the most penetrating, the most powerful intellects.

The word "nature" suggests something different to different persons. Not long since, the study of nature was all but confined to the non-sentient world, the world outside the perceiving mind of man. After Descartes and Locke, philosophers separated sharply the physical and the mental worlds. A new and vigorous assault is in progress, destined to illuminate this old doctrine of the separateness of mind and body. Nature now includes several of its aspects. It means the physical world—the solid, touchable, outside world. But it means also this other world with which critical philosophers are again beginning to be concerned, namely, that world of the mind which seems to lie outside of, and actually to escape, the will but which, nevertheless, is accessible to experience and appears in fact to be that part of the mental apparatus in which experience, often completely forgotten, is stored. This is its aspect which so often presents to us the *faits accomplis* of its own activity, often to our amazement and often also to our delight. This function of the whole human organism is also a phase of nature. When, as now, the need arises to bridge the seeming duality of human nature, and no longer to keep the two worlds of the body and of the mind apart, separateness ceases to be either so decisive or so much a fact as for nearly three centuries it seemed to be. Nature is again mainly of two sorts; non-living and living. And the living world is now once more, the mind and the body. Science as well as art, which confined so long their interests practically and exclusively to the physical, outside world, both have turned again an interested eye inward toward that storehouse and its operations which is the mind.

An enumeration which includes *Kubla Khan,* the *Last Judgment* in the Sistine Chapel, the Theorem of Least Action, the Laws of Mendelian Inheritance, *St. John of Siena,* the First Law of Thermodynamics, the equations describing electromagnetic induction, the circulation of the blood, and the *Ninth Symphony* is a bald catalogue from which those similarities and dissimilarities between art and science which I intend to test cannot possibly emerge, certainly at the beginning of this essay. Obviously, the way out of this apparently unresolvable complex is to arrange these heterogeneous objects into orders which have congruity and so become susceptible to some sort of analysis.

Though this discussion is by no means new, it has fallen into confusion because of the failure to distinguish sharply between persons, artists and scientists on the one hand; and those abstract subjects, art and science, on the other. Passing from art to an artist and from science to a scientist is in practice so frequent and so fluid that it is small wonder the two have been so bewilderingly and blunderingly confused with consequent unfortunate results. Scientists and artists are themselves capable of committing this error. It is no uncommon experience to meet with a scientist who believes that, because he has succeeded in developing an insight into some natural phenomenon, his discovery is equivalent to a vested interest. He has identified his intervention with nature itself. He has converted an observer into a possessor.

Nor is this the only confusion; there is an associated one. It deals with the matter of scientific systems. Observers often are caught believing that because two things absorb their interest, these two belong somehow systematically together. It is as if a sculptor being interested in plants, believed that this interest somehow made him a botanist; and that if he were by chance a teacher, he could teach botany instead of modeling. It seems absurd, but I have known this transposition to take place and in a serious discussion the attempt made to justify it. Personally, both may be his concern. But systematically sculpture does not belong to botany. The error is like the error of the poetic fallacy. A thing, being a thing in its own right, does not become something else because of the chance interest of an interloping admirer.

"Artist" and "scientist," "art" and "science" are terms which should awake vastly different connotations. The basic difference between artists and scientists presumably results from a difference in endowment, a congenital, perhaps an inherited matter. If birth provides men with different natures are their capabilities to be cultivated in different ways? And what may they be? How is a painting conceived or an experiment undertaken? Is what goes on in the minds of these two kinds of persons, during creation, the same or different? An analysis of these matters falls in the domain of biography and specifically in the province of that form of biography, which is essentially a study in psychology. I intend presently to investigate the difference between artists and scientists, but first to inquire into the nature of art and science.

II. ART AND SCIENCE

To define the proper domains of art and science is a systematic enterprise, possible to the discursive reason, interesting to a few persons, but to many men, a dry business.

To say that the object of the two, of science and of art, is similar is to enter upon controversial ground; and to say further that the object of interest in both cases is "nature," does not illuminate the general position. That part of the statement which asserts that the object of interest in science is nature would meet with little opposition. No one doubts that science is concerned with the outside, with the physical world, with what is called "objective reality."

But to know that there is a world of matter and that there are men who are interested in its properties by no means exhausts the statements which can be made about this perplexing subject. Science, having been created by men, has taken on a life of its own, a method which has gradually become suited to its function, proceeding according to carefully tried ways to the accomplishment of its objectives. It has a technique of description of which meticulous accuracy is a foundation and often turns out to be the indispensable keystone of its structure. But description of the physical world, that is only the beginning—description of any part of it indeed, believed for the moment to be interesting, though no one may know at the outset of a scientific enterprise whether it leads to fruitful fields. Who would guess that pursuing the meaning of different results, very slight differences in fact, in the weight of an atom in the third place of decimals would start a train of researches that would end in the explosion of an atomic bomb.

Science

A collection of descriptions, no matter how many there are, is, however, no more usable than the collection of names, *Kubla Khan, St. John of Siena,* the Laws of Mendelian Inheritance which I have recited. A description to be usable must be classifiable. Descriptions dealing with light must be assembled separately; so must those concerning the motions of planets and those which explore the inheritance of morphological characters. The divisions and the subdivisions of separable phenomena have become enormous and are becoming more numerous day by day; to many they begin to appear endless and themselves to issue in nothing but confusion. But even separating groups or classes of phenomena, though interesting—indeed, an essential part of the business—is not the end nor the object of science. Confusion would become merely more refined. The object of science goes further; its intention is to say something definite, as briefly as possible, a short sentence perhaps, summing up the entire meaning, about each set of phenomena. Nor are even these statements the end of the process; they are only the first stage in the art of generalizing or of reasoning. Next comes a stage in which the common factor contained in single statements about two classes—about electricity and about magnetism, for example—is sought in order to make a still more general statement, true of both classes. That is what Clerk-Maxwell managed to do. Newton, to take another instance, observed and analyzed light so that certain phases, common to its various forms, could be jointly described. And recently Einstein has brought together in a single statement—a very simple one, to the elect—the essential conceptions about Clerk-Maxwell's generalization and Newton's generalization. His single statement combining two in the preceding stage, and, in a stage antecedent to this combination, a multiplicity of separate phenomena, represents a triumphant success in scientific enterprise. That is the object of science—to make statements about the world, as few of them, and as brief, as possible, the proof of their value being that they are genuinely descriptive and permit the deepest possible insight into its processes.

Helmholtz, as well as other scientists before and after him, was acutely aware of the significance of this process. He says:

We now come to those sciences which, in respect of the kind of intellectual labour they require, stand at the opposite end of the series to philology and history; namely, the natural and physical sciences. I do not mean to say that in many branches even of these sciences an instinctive appreciation of analogies and a certain artistic sense have no part to play. On the contrary, in natural history the decision which characteristics are to be looked upon as important for classification, and which as unimportant, what divisions of the animal and vegetable kingdoms are more natural than others, is really left to an instinct of this kind, acting without any strictly definable rule. And it is a very suggestive fact that it was an artist, Goethe, who gave the first impulse to the researches of comparative anatomy into the analogy of corresponding organs in different animals, and to the parallel theory of the metamorphosis of leaves in the vegetable kingdom; and thus, in fact, really pointed out the direction which the science has followed ever since. But even in those departments of science where we have to do with the least understood vital processes it is, speaking generally, far easier to make out general and comprehensive ideas and principles, and to express them in definite language, than in cases where we must base our judgment on the analysis of the human mind. It is only when we come to the experimental sciences to which mathematics are applied, and especially when we come to pure mathematics, that we see the peculiar characteristics of the natural and physical sciences fully brought out.[1]

[1] H. Helmholtz, *Popular Lectures on Scientific Subjects*. Translated by E. Atkinson, New York, 1873, p. 20.

A work of art will turn out to be very different. There will be not general, but concrete, individual expressions of a special outlook on the eternal appearances of nature, peculiar to *each* artist, their value residing precisely in the distinctiveness of his view and insight.[2] There will be not *single* statements corresponding to descriptions of the few basic processes which go on in nature, true or intended to be true for all time—but *many,* as many indeed as there are seeing eyes and feeling souls and deft narrators of the countless phenomena and illusions in nature, come upon by the sensitive perceptions of men.

From the objective of science the *method* of science must be sharply distinguished. The method is the procedure which permits scientists to make those statements which have just been discussed. The method is the reverse of objective. If the objective is to condense, to pull many statements into one or as few as possible, the method pulls nature apart so as to view each of the parts separately. Light, for example, is studied separately from electricity, and heat separately from mechanics; the circulation of the blood is described separately from the respiration, the contraction of muscles separately from digestion. This process goes on and on, down to cells in living plants and animals and down to electrons, positrons and neutrons in atoms and to the relations among them. Each function of the organism, isolated from the whole organism, is separately studied; and the statements about each are arranged each after its kind, so that the general state-

[2] "I cannot teach my art, nor the art of any school, since I deny that art can be taught, or, in other words, maintain that art is completely individual, and that the talent of each artist is but the result of his own inspiration and his own study of past tradition. I add that, in my opinion, art or talent, for an artist, is merely a means of applying his personal faculties to the ideas and the things of the period in which he lives.

In particular, the art of painting can consist only in the representation of objects visible and tangible to the painter. An epoch can be reproduced only by its own artists. I mean by the artists who have lived in it. I hold that the artists of one century are fundamentally incompetent to represent the things of a past or future century—in other words, to paint the past or the future.

"It is in this sense that I deny the existence of an historical art applied to the past. Historical art is by its very nature contemporary."—Gustave Courbet in *Artists on Art,* edited by R. Goldwater and M. Treves, New York, 1945, p. 295.

ments already mentioned can then be made. This method of pulling apart and examining in detail is the process of analysis; analysis is the distinguishing, the characteristic, the fundamental method of science. There was a hope, entertained not so long ago and still entertained by many persons, that, an organism having been pulled apart and lying about in pieces, like Humpty Dumpty, it would be possible, once having understood how the machine is made, to fit it together again. This is the hope of the scientific enterprise in the effort of synthesizing the separated, or separate, parts. The end of this process was to culminate in a state of complete knowledge, complete understanding. But, as in the case of Humpty Dumpty, fitting the parts together again later has proved both an illusive and an elusive enterprise. Elusive because, though the search has been energetic, it has rarely, as a matter of fact, been accomplished in really important connections; [3] and illusive because something beyond what is expected occurs when two seemingly unrelated things are put or come together. The enterprise is like pressing the button of jack-in-the-box; if you come untutored to the experience, the last thing you expect to happen is the emergence of Jack. He represents the unpredictable, the incalculable factor in the new adventure. He is what the philosophers call "emergent," and the doctrine which his coming illustrates is the doctrine of "emergent evolution."

Science understands by analyzing, by accumulating its analyses, and by making general statements, the most general possible about experience. The adventure of science is the enterprise which proposes to understand the mechanism of nature—to say inescapable and incontrovertible truths about her performances. As incidental to understanding, the path becomes open for the attempt to convert its operations into use for the benefit of man. Illumination with electricity demonstrates a success to which the use of the plan can triumphantly point. There can be no doubt that by the

---

[3] The ultimate subdivisions of cells and atoms seem to be known. But between finished products and ultimate constituents there are unconnected, intermediate levels of organization, each playing a role. The precise level is decisive for behavior. How and when, if a given behavior is unwanted, interference is to occur, forms the artistic side, to be discussed later, of the scientific enterprise.

method of science, certain of the many aspects of nature can be comprehended and certain of its forces can be controlled.

The Arts

What the objects of science and its methods are can be described with a certain assurance. The objects and the methods of art are, on the other hand, far more difficult to define. Being less specific more, many more, divergent views demand a hearing. Art, all the arts, are concerned with some aspect of nature,[4] but the phase of it which comes into play is necessarily different from that which is conspicuous in science. Helmholtz dealt also with this problem.

Though I have maintained that it is in the physical sciences, and especially in such branches of them as are treated mathematically, that the solution of scientific problems has been most successfully achieved, you will not, I trust, imagine that I wish to depreciate other studies in comparison with them. If the natural and physical sciences have the advantage of great perfection in form, it is the privilege of the moral sciences to deal with a richer material, with questions that touch more nearly the interests and the feelings of man, with the human mind itself, in fact, in its motives and the different branches of its activity. They have, indeed, the loftier and the more difficult task, but yet they cannot afford to lose sight of the example of their rivals, which, in form at least, have, owing to the more ductile nature of their materials, made greater progress.[5]

The moral sciences, by not a large stretch may be made to include the arts. In art, it is as well for the moment, to lose sight of the example of "their rivals." The mere analytical facts of nature may not have an interest for art, though it is precisely the

[4] The writings of artists in the past few centuries leave no doubt that for most of them there was full acceptance of this view. "Wouldn't it be better to soak yourself in nature? I don't hold the view that we have been fooling ourselves and rightly should worship the steam engine, with the great majority. No, a thousand times no! We are here to show the way! According to you salvation lies with the primitives, the Italians. According to me this is incorrect. Salvation lies in nature, now more than ever."—Camille Pissarro, in *Artists on Art*, edited by R. Goldwater and M. Treves, New York, 1945, p. 319.

[5] *Op. cit.*, pp. 24-25.

belief that they do which Mr. John W. Beatty [6] is at pains to demonstrate in a series of quotations from painters and sculptors themselves. The view has in fact been advocated that, even if accurate representation may once have been an essential function of painting and sculpture, photography has come to relieve it of this burden.[7] When it is said in our day that art has become free, this must mean free to see the world, not meticulously or metrically, but as it actually looks to the discerning eye of an interested beholder. The eye of a beholder cannot by any stretch

[6] *The Relation of Art to Nature,* New York, 1922.

[7] This, as a matter of fact, seems to me to be the more tenable view. See also W. M. Ivins, Jr., "Photography and the 'Modern' Point of View: A Speculation in the History of Taste," *Metropolitan Museum Studies,* I, 1928, p. 16. It can also, as in Mr. Beatty's case, be amply supported. Maritain supplies this evidence: "The imitative arts do not aim at copying the appearance of Nature, nor at portraying 'the ideal,' but at making a beautiful object by manifesting a *form* with the help of sensible signs" (J. Maritain, *The Philosophy of Art,* Ditchling, Sussex, 1923, p. 90). And he adds later: "Art then remains at bottom essentially constructive and creative. It is the faculty of producing, doubtless not out of nothing, but out of pre-existing matter, a new creature, an original being, capable on its own part of stirring the soul of a man. This new creature is the fruit of a spiritual marriage, which conjoins the activity of the artist to the passivity of a given material" (*op. cit.,* p. 91).

And "Maurice Denis for his part," quotes Maritain, "stated in perfectly correct terms the same truth, when he wrote:—'Recollect that a picture, before being any sort of anecdote, is in essence a plane surface covered over with colours put together in a given

order'" (*Art et Critique,* August 23, 1890).

"Again, Cézanne said: 'I wanted to copy Nature, I did not get so far. But I was pleased with myself when I found out that the sun, for instance, could not be *reproduced,* but had to be *represented* by something else . . . by colour'" (Maurice Denis, *Theories*).

"'You must not paint from Nature,'" said in his turn in a sally which needs understanding that scrupulous observer of nature, M. Degas (a saying related by J. E. Blanche, *De David á Degas*).

"'In fact,' remarks Baudelaire, 'all good draughtsmen and true draw from the image in their brain and not from Nature. If you adduce the admirable sketches of Raphael, Watteau, and many others, we say they are notes, very detailed it is true, but still mere notes. When a true artist has arrived at the actual execution of his work, the model would be to him more a hindrance than a help. . . .'" (Maritain, p. 151).

"Gaugin and Maurice Denis, for instance, artists who (like many others in the 'young school') are very scrupulous thinkers, will tell you that 'what is most to be deplored . . . is the idea that Art is the *copy* of something' (*Theories,* p. 28); to think that Art consists in copying or exactly reproducing things is to pervert the meaning of Art (*ibid.,* p. 36)" (Maritain, p. 153).

"Ingres, on the contrary, or Rodin, more passionate and less keen of under-

of the imagination be regarded as disinterested.[8] As a matter of fact, that this is possible was never believed to be true, though it is no exaggeration to claim for our own time the introduction of the right to see with our minds and through our own eyes. This is perhaps a correct view, because, though in times past, people learned through their own senses, the *right* to do so came gradually and only, as the Impressionists have insisted, as the result of revolt. This has been the case in art, in science, in politics—in everything, in fact, which distinguishes the present from former social conceptions. The difference between *fact* and *right* makes a difference. The difference may be in degree only, and not a difference in kind. Something is gained though in sharpening the argument so that kind rather than degree is adopted as the point of view.

If artists use their unsupported, naïve senses as the media through which they observe nature, it is precisely because this is their method, that what issues is different from the data of science. "The painter who draws merely by practise and by the eye, with-

standing, will tell you that you must 'copy quite earnestly, quite dully, you must copy servilely, what is before your eyes.' (Amaury-Duval, *L'atelier d' Ingres.*) 'In all things obey nature and never pretend to command her. My only ambition is to be servilely faithful to her' (Paul Gsell, *Rodin*). . . ." (Maritain, p. 154).

"M. Ingres, as M. Denis so judiciously makes clear (*Theories*, pp. 86-98), intended to copy the beauty *which he discerned in nature by going to* the Greeks and Raphael; 'he thought,' says Amaury-Duval, 'that he was copying nature for us in copying her as he saw her'; and he was the first to 'make monsters' according to the saying of Odilon Redon" (Maritain, p. 124).

"'If I have altered anything from nature,' said Rodin, 'it was without any misgiving at the moment. The feeling which influenced my vision showed me nature just as I have copied her. . . . If I had wanted to modify what

I saw and make it more beautiful, I would have turned out nothing good' (J. E. Blanche, *Propos de Peintre, de David à Degas*)" (Maritain, p. 156).

"One cannot insist too much in this connection on the distinction already pointed out . . . between 'the vision' of the artist or his invention, his *conception* of the work, and the *means* of execution or of realisation which he uses. On the side of vision or conception, ingenuousness, spontaneity, candour, which is unconscious of itself, is the artist's most precious gift; a gift unique and preeminent, which Goethe looked upon as 'daemonic,' so much it seemed to him gratuitous and beyond analysis" (Maritain, p. 159).

[8] ". . . *art* seems to stray from the true direction, which is the return to *nature*. For we have to approach nature sincerely, with our own modern sensibilities.—Camille Pissarro, in *Artists on Art*, edited by R. Goldwater and M. Treves, New York, 1945, p. 318.

out any reason, is like a mirror which copies everything placed in front of it without being conscious of their existence," said Leonardo.[9] It would be to labor an argument should one set out elaborately to show that if the same senses of vision, of hearing, of touch, are necessarily used both in science and in art, it is, so far as science is concerned, absolutely requisite to maintain the primary (Galilean) qualities of objects in a state of purity, scrupulously uncontaminated by their secondary or accidental qualities, such as "colours, sounds, odours, tastes, heat, hardness," [10] those impure qualities which, as everyone knows, are of irreplaceable and inalienable value in art—the very qualities indeed which make art possible.

With the passage of time, art has depended more and more on the "strain of impurity." This emphasis has triumphed, so that now it is the general view that of the two qualities of an object, primary and secondary, or pure and impure, or unadulterated description by the senses and adjusted interpretation by the mind, the process of interpretation is the more important.

The point, it must now be clear, is that if nature is the concern of art, it is not the nature of science, nor nature naïvely perceived by the senses, but nature vastly modified and made sophisticated by the use which the emotions and by the interpretations which the reflective mind place on the original experience. Without man his tensions, his searchings and his vagaries, there is no art, though without us nature will still continue to operate according to what are described as nature's laws. Art, to please us, must endow nature with value; and value, being what it is, fluctuates with all the variety to which passion has made men heir.

It is precisely because of the human nature of man that he has turned nature to the use of his emotional requirements. Nature in the great variety of its manifestations is his familiar home. He has learned to utilize these very manifestations as the symbols of his emotions until they have become so much matters of conven-

[9] *The Literary Works of Leonardo da Vinci*, compiled by Jean Paul Richter. London, 1883, I, p. 18.

[10] R. Descartes, Sixth Meditation, quoted by A. N. Whitehead in *Science and the Modern World*, New York, 1925, p. 76.

tion that a thing may actually stand for a feeling. To what extent men have at times ceased to regard nature in any but a symbolic form is apparent in Byzantine art. Its creators, so much more concerned with making immanent their philosophical objectives than is observable in naturalistic representation, actually chose, after much modification, the form they employed, not for the form's sake, but aggressively to suggest the ideas, the thoughts, and the feelings they intended that these should convey. It seems almost necessary to conclude, since a wealth of naturalistic Greco-Roman art then so recently in its heyday had survived (its remains lying in profusion all about the Aegean litoral), and since their technical skill apparently was adequate to their needs, that the abstract, symbolic forms they employed must have had their origin in ulterior motives rather than in a desire or need merely to imitate nature. It is another of the exhibitions of the sophisticated, selective behavior of men—this use of nature for edification rather than for representation. Nor is Byzantine art the only example of the employment of nature for the purpose of edification. Only recently Mr. Cram has been telling us that

here lies the province of art where it has ever lain; for in all its manifestations, whether as architecture, painting, sculpture, drama, poetry, or ritual, it is the only visible and concrete expression of this mystical power in man which is greater than physical force, greater than physical mind, whether with M. Bergson we call it intuition or with Christian philosophers we call it the immortal soul.[11]

And he says later:

[The artist], Master of the great language, articulate among the tongueless, it is for him to express all the spiritual essays, ventures, and discoveries; all the dreams, aspirations, and visions of the mounting wave of humanity that bears him on its crest toward the stars. Seer, spokesman, and prophet, he divines in scientific triumphs the inner significance that gives them value and that the scientist himself sometimes sees not at all.[12]

[11] R. A. Cram, *The Ministry of Art,*   [12] *Ibid,* p. 111.
Boston and New York, 1914, p. 8.

Enough has now been said to make manifest the functions of art in respect to nature; to represent, to be the language and the expression of the emotions, to serve the purpose of symbolic representation of the great and good life. Great art, in great epic poetry, has achieved still another success and supplied still another need. It has in the *Aeneid,* in the *Divine Comedy* and in *Paradise Lost,* constructed entire cosmologies and symbolical epitomes of their histories for the use of their respective cultures. In his invocation Milton requests the muse to

> Sing . . . .
> . . . who first taught the chosen seed,
> In the beginning how the Heavens and Earth
> Rose out of Chaos: . . .

And he begs the

> Spirit, that dost prefer
> Before all temples the upright heart and pure,
> Instruct me, for thou know'st; . . . .
> . . . . What in me is dark,
> Illumine; what is low, raise and support;
> That to the highth of this great argument
> I may assert Eternal Providence,
> And justify the ways of God to men.

In this large and wide-embracing view the great epics have sought to serve the very function of science. In employing the vast resources of poetry they, the ultimate flowers of their culture, have succeeded in sublimating the beliefs, developed in their cultures, on the ways of nature, and in the end have been the means of indoctrinating them as dogma. It would be idle to contend gravely that either in intention or in method does their purpose parallel the aim of science. Their mood is neither inquiring nor speculative. Their wisdom is the wisdom which issues from approved beliefs. The purpose is declaration and criticism.

Music

These assertions should be examined in the case of each art sufficiently at least to test the thesis. Music, being the most general, comes first; it is the simplest and purest of the arts. If it has a quality at all characteristic of the physical world, it is time. Narration gives music its sense of duration, a different, and another, sense of time from that connected with the dance. The need was to exteriorize or to express emotions which lie deep buried in the nature of primitive, and quite clearly also of later sophisticated mankind. Nor has music exhausted this primitive strain. It has learned instead to develop its range and to increase the complexity of its utterance. No one sensitive to its expressiveness can doubt its fast-deepening and ever more varied content, during the past two centuries, of human emotion.

Its language is, nevertheless, the most, and at the same time, the least familiar of the arts. It is the least familiar because, being without measurable dimensions, it is uncolored and unaided by those accessories of experience which spoken language and vision supply. Hearing, in a primitive sense, gives an account of a limited gamut of experience, only. So deprived, it is the most restricted of the arts. It is, on the other hand, the most familiar, because there is scarce a phase of the emotional life, which it is unable to express. Those who know its language can communicate in music with extraordinary directness and simplicity the most profound feelings of which men are capable, and can convey them, in their pure state, in a way which surpasses the resources of the other arts. It is the most direct in the authentic expression of emotional experience. The current attempt to deepen the range and to make us, through hearing, responsive to the growing complexity of contemporary life, no doubt strains the idiom and makes its immediate appreciation more difficult. But the effort, it appears, continues nevertheless to be made.

The recognition in music of its predominantly emotional expressiveness leaves in an equivocal position a relation which it once held to mathematics, as when the Pythagoreans and later

152 No Retreat from Reason

Greeks were interested in both, and were especially concerned to see in number certain correspondences with the physical world. Formal Greek education included both music and mathematics; and the medieval curriculum, combined music with arithmetic, geometry, and astronomy—all mathematical disciplines—in the quadrivium. It has been observed that men in whom a mathematical sense is singularly developed turn easily and eagerly to music. Mr. J. W. N. Sullivan is an example. At mathematical congresses the claims of music are said to make striking inroads upon the organized proceedings. The question is natural, therefore, whether music and mathematics do not possess a similarity which makes their association fitting and perhaps inevitable. The essential factor can scarcely be recurrence and rhythm, for poetry also possesses these. An analysis having greater statistical virtue would be valuble in establishing these speculations more firmly. At the same time Dr. Buchanan professes to see in poetry, a comparable relation.[13] But the problem is complex because in a strict sense mathematics is not, as are physics and physiology, a natural science.

This is a knotty problem for which the time is not ripe to attempt a solution. The difficulty certainly has been: What is the earmark of an emotion—of fear, of love, or pleasure—as expressed in music,[14] and how can it be recognized? Is what Mr. Sullivan experiences in Beethoven's last quartets clearly apparent to other men, presumably as understanding of musical utterance as was he? Obviously, this is not the fact. The door lies open for an important further exploration in sensitiveness to this form of experience.

Poetry

Epic, narrative, dramatic poetry exploit a physical dimension, time. Lyric poetry is naturally to be dissociated from its fellows; having its origin in emotion, and being an expression of a mood. In its interpretative quality resides the value of poetry. But there are two further orders of poetry. Of the poetry of devotion noth-

[13] *Poetry and Mathematics,* New York, 1929.

[14] J. W. N. Sullivan, *Beethoven, His Spiritual Development,* London, 1927.

ing need be added to the quotation from Mr. Cram.[15] But there is the well-known case of "pure poetry" to which Mr. Herbert Read has again devoted attention in a recent essay.[16] Pure poetry depends, and is intended to depend, for its effect upon the choice and sound of words, apart entirely from the meaning to which their pattern gives rise. *Kubla Khan* is such a poem. Pure poetry delights us because of its limpidness, its fluidity, the musical quality of its phrase, the suggestiveness of individual words, but not necessarily their meaning. This poetry serves a subtler function. It sets resonating a complex of emotions. It releases tension. This is a poet's opportunity to deal exquisitely with human nature; here a knowledge of her processes is the clue to utilizing suitable instruments to gain appointed ends. To succeed, an experiment must be carefully calculated. Coleridge is an admirable witness:

During the first year that Mr. Wordsworth and I were neighbors, our conversations turned frequently on the two cardinal points of poetry, the power of exciting the sympathy of the reader by a faithful adherence to the truth of nature, and the power of giving the interest of novelty by the modifying colors of imagination. The sudden charm which accidents of light and shade, which moonlight or sunset diffused over a known and familiar landscape, appeared to represent the practicability of combining both. These are the poetry of nature. The thought suggested itself—(to which of us I do not recollect)—that a series of poems might be composed of two sorts. In the one, the incidents and agents were to be, in part at least, supernatural; and the excellence aimed at was to consist in the interesting of the affections by the dramatic truth of such emotions, as would naturally accompany such situations, supposing them real. And real in this sense they have been to every human being who, from whatever source of delusion, has at any time believed himself under supernatural agency. For the second class, subjects were to be chosen from ordinary life; the characters and incidents were to be such as will be found in every village and its vicinity, where there is a meditative and feeling mind to seek after them, or to notice them, when they present themselves.

In this idea originated the plan of the LYRICAL BALLADS; in which

[15] See page 149.   [16] Herbert Read, *Phases of English Poetry*, London, 1928.

it was agreed, that my endeavors should be directed to persons and characters supernatural, or at least romantic; yet so as to transfer from our inward nature a human interest and a semblance of truth sufficient to procure for these shadows of imagination that willing suspension of disbelief for the moment, which constitutes poetic faith. Mr. Wordsworth, on the other hand, was to propose to himself as his object, to give the charm of novelty to things of every day, and to excite a feeling analogous to the supernatural, by awakening the mind's attention to the lethargy of custom, and directing it to the loveliness and the wonders of the world before us; an inexhaustible treasure, but for which, in consequence of the film of familiarity and selfish solicitude we have eyes, yet see not, ears that hear not, and hearts that neither feel nor understand.[17]

The Ancient Mariner, The Darke Ladie, and *Christabel* represent Coleridge's interpretation of this assignment; Wordsworth wrote the *Lyrical Ballads.*

Sculpture and Painting

Sculpture and painting have for long periods followed closely representation of the physical world. Opinion varies greatly on the value of accuracy or of imitation. It is worth remembering the role Leonardo and Michelangelo played in the return to naturalism. Leonardo and later Calcar were forerunners; the anatomists, Vesalius for example, were successors. They would have come along, no doubt, but the actual sequence lends an important insight into how "progress" is made. Professionals in a discipline do not always lead. How far away and conservative the day seems when Lessing wrote: "Painting, as now carried out in its whole compass, may be defined generally as the art of imitating figures on a *flat* surface; . . ."[18] And also: "I believe the fact, that it is *to a single moment* that the material limits of art confine all its imitations, will lead us to similar views."[19] In sculp-

[17] S. T. Coleridge, Complete works. *Biographia Literaria.* New York, 1884, p. 364.
[18] G. E. Lessing, *Selected Prose*

Works. Translated by E. C. Beasley and Helen Zimmern, London, 1890, p. 11. The italics are mine.
[19] *Ibid.,* p. 19.

ture it is not to a flat surface, but to a volume, to which these observations apply. To Lessing it seemed obvious, and it did so to many critics both then and since, that the representation of an object, in painting or in sculpture, be confined to a single moment, an *instant of time*. If formerly bi-dimensional and tri-dimensional representation were instantaneous—caught frozen in a moment of time—to sculptors like Brancusi and to a school of Cubists, the introduction of a further element, time, not previously regarded as proper to the graphic arts, has become commonplace. How else can the flight of a bird be regarded when carved in marble than as a four-dimensional figure? And how otherwise than as tri-dimensional, a collection of objects on a canvas, fragments of a fiddle, of a vase, of a table, as if, consequent on the rotation of one's head, persistent retinal after-images were reproduced on canvas after having been observed in succession by an artist's eye? Here after Lessing, is something new—not scrupulous selection so as to exclude the intrusion of time, but the representation of time itself.

The conviction has grown furthermore that freer revelation of events in the intimate history of the lives of persons is desirable. This is not the critical analysis of simple, moral situations, as in Daumier and Hogarth, but the description of images as they occur in dreams or in day-dreams, in the effort to communicate events that are taking place in one's unconscious life. It is a far cry, this, from the simpler day of Lessing.

Enough evidence has now been accumulated to connect in several ways the arts first with the material, physical world, and then with their ever-deepening responsiveness to the views, the emotions, the complex mental life of man.[20]

It is often said that, if it is the function of science to attempt to understand the operations of nature by the method of analysis, it is the function of art to perform a like office by the method of synthesis. This statement contains either confusion of conception or else insufficient description of what is meant by "synthesis." If by synthesis is meant that the creation of a completed work

---

[20] Another relation of graphic art to science is discussed in the essay on *The* *Influence of Modern Science on Painting and Sculpture*, p. 42.

of art depends on knowledge of an object by dissecting that object first into its component parts and later by reassembling the fragments, there may be ground for the idea. That this has been the process is, however, not detectable in a finished work. As a matter of fact, it is doubtful whether a synthesis of constituent parts is consciously made except possibly by early cubists. "Consciously" is important, for if the synthesis takes place in one's unconscious, it is no synthesis in any usual sense. If it has taken place as an extra conscious operation, the situation is different, as I intend presently to show. However an artist arrives at the idea of his creation, this much is clear, that he cannot hope to incarnate a living world unless he himself has experienced and felt that world in its emotional wholeness. And he must reproduce it as he himself has experienced or conceived it; otherwise it will disintegrate before a critical scrutiny. If, to one thing more than to another, an observer is sensitive, it is this quality of unity. This is the characteristic which makes of a work of art something else than the recollected disjointed elements of an experience.

These two passages from Proust are extraordinarily eloquent statements on the wholeness of a work of art, which cannot, it seems, be synthetic if in the course of its birth it has never been analytic.

. . . for then Vinteuil, seeking to do something new, questioned himself, with all the force of his creative effort, reached his own essential nature at those depths, where whatever be the question asked, it is in the same accent, that is to say its own, that it replies. Such an accent, the accent of Vinteuil, is separated from the accents of other composers by a difference far greater than that which we perceive between the voices of two people, even between the cries of two species of animal: by the difference that exists between the thoughts of these other composers and the eternal investigations of Vinteuil, the question that he put to himself in so many forms, his habitual speculation, but as free from analytical formulas of reasoning as if it were being carried out in the world of the angels, so that we can measure its depth, but without being any more able to translate it into human speech than are disincarnate spirits when, evoked by a medium, he questions them as to the mysteries of death . . .

This lost country composers do not actually remember, but each of them remains all his life somehow attuned to it; he is wild with joy when he is singing the airs of his native land, betrays it at times in his thirst for fame, but then, in seeking fame, turns his back upon it, and it is only when he despises it that he finds it when he utters, whatever the subject with which he is dealing, that peculiar strain the monotony of which—for whatever its subject it remains identical in itself—proves the permanence of the elements that compose his soul. But is it not the fact then that from those elements, all the real residuum which we are obliged to keep to ourself, which cannot be transmitted in talk, even by friend to friend, by master to disciple, by lover to mistress, that ineffable something which makes a difference in quality between what each of us has felt and what he is obliged to leave behind at the threshold of the phrases in which he can communicate with his fellows only by limiting himself to external points common to us all and of no interest, art, the art of a Vinteuil like that of an Elstir, makes the man himself apparent, rendering externally visible in the colours of the spectrum the intimate composition of those worlds which we call individual persons and which, without the aid of art, we should never know. A pair of wings, a different mode of breathing, which would enable us to traverse infinite space, would in no way help us, for, if we visited Mars or Venus keeping the same senses, they would clothe in the same aspect as the things of the earth everything that we should be capable of seeing. The only true voyage of discovery, the only fountain of Eternal Youth, would be not to visit strange lands but to possess other eyes, to behold the universe through the eyes of another, of a hundred others, to behold the hundred universes that each of them beholds, that each of them is; and this we can contrive with an Elstir, with a Vinteuil; with men like these we do really fly from star to star.[21]

Proust is speaking here of music; but an exactly comparable train of reflection flows from Coleridge's description of poetry. His use of the word "synthesis" differs from the one I have been discussing. Joined with the word "magical," it obviously denotes a process akin to intuition, a function to be analyzed in greater detail later.

[21] M. Proust, *The Captive*. Translated by C. K. Scott Moncrieff, New York, 1929, p. 346-47.

My own conclusions on the nature of poetry, in the strictest use of the word, have been in part anticipated in some of the remarks on the Fancy and Imagination in the first part of this work. What is poetry? is so nearly the same question with, What is a poet?—that the answer to the one is involved in the solution of the other. For it is a distinction resulting from the poetic genius itself, which sustains and modifies the images, thoughts, and emotions of the poet's own mind.

The poet, described in ideal perfection, brings the whole soul of man into activity, with the subordination of its faculties to each other according to their relative worth and dignity. He diffuses a tone and spirit of unity, that blends, and (as it were) *fuses*, each into each, by that synthetic and magical power, to which I would exclusively appropriate the name of Imagination. This power, first put in action by the will and understanding, and retained under their irremissive, though gentle and unnoticed, control, *laxis effertur habenis*, reveals itself in the balance or reconcilement of opposite or discordant qualities: of sameness, with difference; of the general with the concrete; the idea with the image; the individual with the representative; the sense of novelty and freshness with old and familiar objects; a more than usual state of emotion with more than usual order; judgment ever awake and steady self-possession with enthusiasm and feeling profound or vehement; and while it blends and harmonizes the natural and the artificial, still subordinates art to nature; the manner to the matter; and our admiration of the poet to our sympathy with the poetry. . . .

Finally, Good Sense is the Body of poetic genius, Fancy its Drapery, Motion its Life, and Imagination the Soul that is everywhere, and in each; and forms all into one graceful and intelligent whole.[22]

The difference between science and art consists not in different methods of descriptions so much as in representing quite different viewpoints of nature. These are not slight but fundamental and profound. In discussing matters in the realm of belief, Richards refers to this problem in its intellectual and emotional phases.

But this intellectual disbelief does not imply that emotional belief in the same idea is either impossible or even difficult—much less that it is undesirable. For an emotional belief is not justified through any logical relations between its idea and other ideas. Its only justification

[22] S. T. Coleridge, *op. cit.*, p. 373.

is its success in meeting our needs—due regard being paid to the relative claims of our many needs one against another. It is a matter, to put it simply, of the *prudence* (in view of *all* the needs of our being) of the kind of emotional activities the belief subserves. The desirability or undesirability of an emotional belief has nothing to do with its intellectual status, provided it is kept from interfering with the intellectual system. And poetry is an extraordinarily successful device for preventing these interferences from arising.[23]

The difference which these two human interests serve is the world of reason, which is science; and the world of art, which is concrete feeling and emotion. If science accomplishes its purpose, which is generalization by analysis, it is the opportunity of art to attain its own, by seeking to awaken a mood and, having done so, sympathetically to convey deep-felt experience by expression. The methods which they employ and the things they say, are as strikingly opposite as are the needs to which they appeal and which they have been called forth to satisfy. It would be extraordinary indeed, were men, so distinguished for the variety of their requirements, content with a single approach only, to understanding the mystery of existence. Their explorations, it is apparent, may not be told in a single way, for a single way does not exhaust the possibilities.

It is a matter of considerable interest, though, to notice that each, art and science, varying with its essence, is influenced by the *Zeitgeist*, and each so as to suggest that the quality of the *Zeitgeist* may be recognized by considering the two together, as it could not have been by the study of each alone. An illustration can be found in that period of any culture which is sensitively expressive of that culture. Our own time may serve as a suitable example. It is characteristic of the past forty years, that there exists a vastly deeper insight into the difference between appearance and reality than was possible in the 17th Century. Atoms, as is now believed, and consequently all matter, which they compose, are no longer regarded as made of "solid" substance; and even this solid substance, is far from being as solid as has

23 I. A. Richards, *Practical Criticism,*
New York, 1929, p. 276.

been supposed. The realization of this discovery has clearly had far-reaching consequences, both in physical theory and in critical philosophy. This reflection has a relevance in painting; a doubt as to the reality of appearance has come to stimulate the imagination. It has taken two forms: one which in cubism has sought to discern, an underlying structure by a new way of visualizing, through a comprehensive analysis of various aspects behind the specious unity (or validity) of a single profile. The other form is to be found in the adventures of those who followed in the pathway of post-impressionism, that is to say abstractionism. Here the performance transcends the views of ordinary simple geometrical form and endows reality with an appearance which it puts many of us at pains to recognize. Examples are to be found in those studies of Picasso in which he has rearranged the features of a face, presumably in order to secure heightened emotional response which a natural arrangement, as such, falls short of stimulating. An artist's purpose and the public assent are deadlocked here. Whether ventures like this are to succeed, seems still to be undecided. In sculpture and poetry, similar tendencies are observable. They are less readily observed in architecture; in music, a younger art, current happenings seem to be attributable to other motives.

The Dance

Of all the "arts" dancing is, with music, the elemental emotional form. It is, furthermore, peculiarly striking how, of successive cultures each is distinguished by a dance pattern of its own. In civilized societies, perhaps in barbaric societies as well, congruity between cultural level and bodily expression is exhibited in a high degree—exquisitely in France in the art of Watteau. The dancing in his scenes is impressive in its satisfying togetherness. No Maenad would feel at home in one of them. Contrariwise, a Maenad would no doubt have been expelled. And so would Agnes de Mille's dancers. Now, self-conscious intention has made dancing become an organic part of the action of a play. This dancing is no interlude, no *divertissement*, no play in itself, like a Russian Ballet. This contemporary dancing is just a way of going on with the action. Player gives way to dancer and dancer again to player. This form has meaning because it depends on exteriorizing in vivid motion happenings in the unconscious, often in the conscious, mind.

If these attitudes have had consequences for concepts of physics, they have had consequences also for conceptions concerning the mind. The study of the behavior of the mind seems now to have entered a phase which in the seriousness of the enterprise has not for three centuries been current. None of its manifestations any longer escapes analytical curiosity, and investigation. This curiosity as to its processs is everywhere manifest. In the *impasse* at which certain aspects of physical science have arrived, appeal is insistently made by physicists themselves to the mind's native qualities; and to it, in its naïve state, unsupported by experimental evidence, are referred questions for decision of great importance. I do not wish to enter into these problems further than to point out that, if under such circumstances appeal is made to the mind, it is in order to obtain an estimate of value; and value obviously is judgment without reference to quantity. Now this reference to the mind, of decisions concerning value, is just the use of the mind which art also makes. In current thought, both science and art attribute to the mind, and rely upon, an identical function.

The Audience

If I pass quickly over the part which the audience plays in these adventures, it is not that I am oblivious of the fact that both science and art are enterprises inextricably intertwined in the social matrix. I do so rather because the audience is not the final cause either of the curiosity or of the feeling which germinates in the minds of artists and scientists, but curiosity aroused by nature itself; nor is society responsible for the genesis or the development of special, departmentalized ideas except in so far as all its members possess a common culture. Thinking and feeling cannot escape being private affairs. Their coming into being results, no doubt, from reciprocal stimulation. From one point of view, that of effective initiation, the audience itself is passive, even if its anticipated judgments, its applause, are constantly prominent presences to creators and often anxiously and prayerfully taken into account. It is, as Maritain says,

. . . quite true that Art *results* in arousing in us affective states of mind, but this is not Art's *end* or *aim:* a slight shade of difference, if you like, but one of extreme importance. All is off the lines if we take for the *end* what is only a *joint-result* or *repercussion;* as also if we make of the end itself (the production of a work in which the splendour of a *form* shines out upon proportioned matter) a simple *means* (of evoking in others a state of mind, an emotion).[24]

The audience in any immediate sense is not the responsible source of the life of reason in scientists, nor of the sensibility of artists, nor their power to feel, nor their emotional understanding. Society, as a whole, has a task; but the stake of society is limited to the circumstance that physically it owns the entire collections of works of art and, as individuals, treasures many examples. In our time it originates almost nothing—even in the sense of patron. Here connoisseurship and bourgeois collecting indulge their pleasure and exhibit their gains. From the viewpoint of sensitiveness, the business of collecting is not a disinterested trade. Collectively it has come, again by way of nature and inheritance, on the necessity and on the ability to be artistically creative; but artistic creativeness is not a function of society but of its individual members.

What a spectator or a critic experiences may be identical with what an artist has experienced for, and before, him, in Bosanquet's sense [25] or in Coomaraswamy's or in Sarton's. This is the function of *Einfühlung.* But this is a matter apart again from participating in the creative process. The audience must inevitably be taken for granted. It partakes, no doubt, in the common thinking and feeling which is everywhere current. In any case artists and scientists, together with everyone else, share alike in these.

[24] J. Maritain, *op. cit.*, p. 165.   [25] B. Bosanquet, *Three Lectures on Aesthetics,* London, 1915, pp. 111-12.

It has been preferable to inquire first as to the part which fact and appearance play in these activities before going on to the men who are responsible for them. The audience, as a third element, is deeply involved but is necessarily, in the sense just defined, passive.

Livelihood

Proper to a consideration of audiences, is a mundane question, the question of earning a living. To live, requires employment. To be employed can occur in one of three ways only. Artists can paint easel pictures including portraits or their equivalents. Easel painting which became prominent in the Renaissance (had it ever been before in Europe?) is an opportunity for a curious reflection. Easel pictures and small pieces of sculpture being easily movable can become objects of purchase. Tanagra figurines may have served the same purpose as may also the small bronzes in Rome and Pompeii. They can become ornaments and occasions for competition in acquisitive societies. The quick response between creator and purchaser plays an important role in this traffic. The sensitive life and thought of an artist becomes part of a mercantile social system. The opportunity may have been present in the Corinthian ceramic trade and perhaps earlier in Crete. The absence of a suitable material, like canvas, may have limited this variety of endeavor. But on this, the literature is sparse. The motive of these employers has been largely *self-gratification* on the part of the audience. They may adorn public buildings and churches, the object being *self-interest*, making appeals or, on a lower level, propaganda for corporate societies or for the state. They may employ their gifts in the interests of public *instruction*, to inculcate public mores or stimulate pride in national history. Like all making-a-living, its ways are precarious—more precarious than the makers of bathtubs encounter. The plumbers supply more widely felt and better advertised needs. Financial depressions emphasize the financial precariousness of artists. If depressions are unavoidable they serve to increase this unhappy dependence. It is a melancholy subject, this. It were good if it could be ignored.

The Museum

The *Museum,* temple of the Muses, or perhaps only the site of a temple is what the ancient prototype of an art gallery was called in Alexandria. It was a store-house of objects, a seat of instruction, and a place devoted to the advancement of learning. If this is what the Alexandrians supported, there rests no obligation on us to follow in their footsteps. We are free to make of our museums what we choose. At a minimum they exist to attract audiences for some designated purpose. *Motives,* more or less modern, have been incorporated in the institution. They came in with that turn in antiquarianism inherited from the self-conscious Renaissance, hankering for a golden age. A sense for history and nostalgia have now been well-established. But there is a third motive, very troublesome. It is called "appreciation"—appreciation on the part of the public of the works of other, original, creative men. Why this is necessary or who needs to feel it is not specified. The suggestion that it is to be experienced mostly during leisure is irritating. "Appreciating" is what you must do if you want to possess "culture"—"culture" being reserved for the leisured rich, especially women. Unfortunately in this view, appreciation, the thing appreciated, and culture are all regarded as things somehow apart from our ordinary daily lives. That was a fault. David once (1798) attributed to all the French "no natural love for the arts in France, but an artificial taste." [26]

Museums house objects, bi- and tridimensional objects. But what *objects?* The consensus of opinion seems to be, everything which men have made, from kitchen utensils to knights in armor. There is frequently a single criterion only for the admission of a particular object—it must be good, each after its own kind. This formula covers almost everything except painting and sculpture and music. Music is a very special case and the most intricate of all, but painting and sculpture are not far behind.

[26] *Artists on Art,* edited by R. Goldwater and M. Treves, NewYork, 1945, p. 206.

The use and value of *painting* and *sculpture* have been much discussed and occasioned much difference of opinion. The range among artists themselves is almost unbelievable, to say nothing of the professors. The value of *a* painting or of *a* piece of sculpture is subject to caprice, to prejudice, and even to politics. There was the case of Rivera and his portrait of Lenin. The painters alive during the French revolution suffered from these prejudices before him. The commonest requisite though of an object, to justify admission is "beauty." The need to possess this quality seems scarcely ever to have been doubted. "Ugliness," whatever that may be, does nevertheless get into museums. Goya's war pieces, if they are ugly, are examples. Such works are often carried in, nevertheless, on G. B. Shaw's formula—"if it's a good author, it's a good play." The reason for insisting on beauty is no doubt implicit in the conceptions and the "ideals" of a society, what the elders wish that society to know, what the professors wish that society to appreciate, whatever the quality is which gives to a creation a good ticket to its "culture."

In short, there is no guarantee; a thing can get wanted for improper, as well as proper, reasons. It depends on whether the authorities decree that a thing is "beautiful." Naturally there are rules. But that puts "beauty" in an awkward place because thoughtful men have had difficulty, indeed much anguish, in trying to define beauty. And if an object has this supposed quality it becomes an object for acquisitiveness. Since only beauty belongs in museums, modern souls must go there to learn lest they be thought not "cultured," to appreciate what the authorities tell them is beauty and therefore to be "appreciated."

There is no reason for agreeing, however, with what someone else has called beautiful. A good many of us do not like Quatrocento Sienese madonnas nor 16th Century Hindu Sivas. We do not think in that idiom—in fact we regard some Indian conceptions with aversion. "Appreciation" is in short an unhappy load for museums to carry. It alienates people. People would go to museums to look at what suits them but don't, because of a feeling of guilt about other things which they shrink from confessing they can't "appreciate." People have often, young people especially, gone only after a struggle, not understanding why they should like a Byzantine saint.

On this point, clarity—and candor—would work a miracle. Suppose we regarded "appreciation" and beauty and culture as fiddlesticks. Suppose we said there are better reasons than appreciation for going to museums. Suppose we said we go for fun or because of something we want to know about. You may want to see how Cretans dressed, or tossed bulls, or bulls tossed them, and how they lived; or inquire what the Egyptians did about their strange notions of death and the hereafter. And so on, through all the forms that have been invented of graphic description, for illumination, for entertainment, for unpurposeful expression or solely and merely for the purpose of record. Once, in 1929, on the deck of a little steamer riding at anchor on a wonderful April day in the harbor of Candia, a German *gymnasium* teacher was discoursing to his pupils on the Labyrinth. He called it the symbol of a leisure class, a class in the enviable state of needing no objective, no excuse for being, no destination—*Nicht zielbewusst,* he called it. A leisure class could afford not to have a *Ziel.* Cretans, some of them, had already arrived at that blissful state. They were the very ones who could appreciate "art"—they were the ones for whom it was made.

If ever there was a time when this was the mood of museums, repositories of precious things chosen by connoisseurs for appreciation by the leisured, this time of general upheaval, of revaluing values, is seeing its unlamented end. It may now become possible to be robust and tough-minded.

To give expression is an inescapable human want. It is always there, though special circumstances forbid it. It is not true that expression waits on leisure. The need to express does not wait; it is always here and very urgent. It takes on extraordinary forms in the conduct of business, in colored prints by Hiroshiga, in tradesmen's cards in England, in the anatomical drawings of great anatomists like Leonardo; illustrations for fun, for edification, for magic in the caves of the Dordogne or for reverence and religious expression in the temples of Greece. To learn the origins of this culture of ours it is a joy and an exhilaration to resort to

museums because there is where it has become customary to collect and exhibit the expressions and experiences of times now past.

We are grateful to scholars, to archaeologists and curators who
find and arrange what has been saved from ultimate destruction
—for our instruction and entertainment and delight. This is the
historical and the pedagogical side of museums—their most valuable opportunity. Without this it would be difficult to know the
meaning and the accomplishments of our culture or to keep its
elements and its ideas in order. Museums are the picture books
of our history, our culture and our suffering—not only painting
and sculpture, but everything we have rescued and know now
we must put into them.

To include having "fun" is more doubtful. Of course we are
not only learned nor always sad. Fun can mean amusement because an object is strange; it can be entertainment because it
gives satisfaction; it can be anything that releases tension or provides the pleasure of recognition, or a change of scene, or a new
expenditure of energy. Who has not been grateful to a comedian
who makes you laugh. His art transcends all other human services
at that moment. A museum can provide humor, perhaps even
more than it is in the habit of doing. It can let us understand
the jibes and the cynicism and the wit and the deep social con-
science of Daumier and Rowlandson and Hogarth. It may even
help to make clear what humor is. Fun, entertainment, whichever you wish—certainly possible to draftsmen, certainly calculated
to draw audiences to the temple of the arts.

Refreshment of the spirit, as a function, belongs here, with
"fun." It is more vague, but it is a need of thoughtful, contem-
plative citizens, for whom variety and entertainment to maintain
the buoyancy of their spirits are legitimate pastimes. Especially
artisans and artists need this—men who communicate with other
men through a plastic medium, the way thinkers do through books,
writers of tales with other writers of tales. "In my Father's house
are many mansions."

So much for "objects of art"—expression might be a better
term. Objects need space. Museums provide it. That takes care

of the conventional conception of museums. But the case of Music! Music is a form of expression as much a part of our culture as the graphic forms. Music has no home in this country comparable to museums. There is no place to which people can resort as of right to enjoy music. Why should they not be permitted to support music as they do museums, with their own money, paid as taxes? You go to a museum to see an old object many times over or to a modern museum to see a new one. Concerts and the opera do the same by repeating over and over what we want to be familiar with. "Pieces" are frequently repeated by orchestras, at the opera, by individual performers. Why? Contrariwise, who has not been distressed by the jumble of works in conventional programs and been annoyed by the undesired repetition of un-wished-for performances. For them he has often to give up the most intimate, the most eloquent expressions of which his soul had need. The difficulties may be insuperable—to hear only what we wish. It may be more troublesome than to see only what we enjoy. Perhaps it is even a little unreasonable. At the same time a public concert is a cause of real complaint. Communion between a composer and oneself is mostly carried on in public under re-pelling circumstances, at hours of the day often inconvenient, in physical discomfort, in unsuitable clothes, in company often of unsympathetic persons, and at an expense beyond what many a sensitive listener can afford—the very person, no doubt, who most desires and has most need of this sympathetic experience.

It is a difficult and many-sided problem. It cannot wholly be solved. A similarity between music and the graphic arts is not immediately apparent. And yet there is a point at which music is brought into relation with them. Concerts *are* given in museums, but with no regard to theory; and in libraries, as in the Library of Congress. Suppose we say a museum is the proper place for music. Why?—because of the need for repetition. That supplies the entering wedge. In this sense concert halls and the opera have been playing an important role. They are, in essence, museums. The misfortune is that music has found too infrequently only a commercial setting. But music can conceivably be supported from taxes just as museums are, for the delight of the public. Incorporation in museums would be not an unreasonable, not an impossible arrangement. That would put the enjoyment of sight and sound together in a proper and suitable setting—like putting schools of related sciences in universities. The works of old and modern masters need constantly to be repeated to make them familiar like the paintings on the walls. Conductors could then become teachers beside being performers. The performance of a "piece" could then be interrupted in order to analyze its structure. That would be appropriate in the intimacy of the "class room." Age and the value of repetition indicate what similarities between music and the graphic arts give them comparable claims to the use of museums. Music, in short, is to be located in museums.

If this suggestion received widespread acceptance, the possibility of vulgar profit, or loss, would disappear from hearing music just as it has from viewing the graphic arts. Music would cease to be the plaything of business. It would leave the opportunity for commercial traffic to new, advanced, contemporary, perhaps unfamiliar forms of music.

How to provide for oncoming generations is a great responsibility. Perhaps, as in science, livings can be found for those who are trying out their wings, by providing devices like scholarships and fellowships. When they have survived the Ph.D. era and the years beyond, positions as teachers and performers and conductors would give them still further security while their educations and their skills and their compositions are in process of being born and their conceptions and styles developed. The business of earning a living is undoubtedly more difficult in music than in any other of the arts and perhaps as lacking in human dignity as in any career, precisely because in our way of life so many persons live as middle men between composers and their audiences— agents, orchestral performers, labor unions, singers, entrepreneurs, a formidable array of persons and groups of persons who raise the cost of enjoyment and to whom, now, we pay tribute—persons who have contributed almost nothing to the emergence of a "work of art."

To maintain balance, to avoid specialization is one of the important difficulties of our time. The danger is the danger of isolation, of losing contact with other activities which make life comprehensible. One of the developments of professionalism has been the narrowing of interest and sympathy and knowledge. Permitting the organization of society to take on compartmentalization of its interests is to court provincialism. Professor Whitehead has completely apprehended wherein the danger lies:

It produces minds in a groove. Each profession makes progress but it is progress in its own groove. Now to be mentally in a groove is to live in contemplating a given set of abstractions. The groove prevents straying across country, and the abstraction abstracts from something to which no further attention is paid. But there is no groove of abstractions which is adequate for the comprehension of human life.[27]

It would be idle to complain that music is exclusively liable to this danger of separation and loneliness, depending as it does on the sense of hearing alone. Even when the medium of communication is through vision and through the tactile and muscular senses, as in science, the loss that results from isolation, from being spacially too far removed from men who have other but cognate intellectual concerns, at least in important aspects, is known and deplored. In the growth of universities and of institutions for research, whether in pure science or in applied, wherever current urgencies have forced related activities apart, the loss resulting from the absence of cross fertilization is acutely felt and much regretted.

It goes without saying that here there is involved a practical matter. Even if all life is one, in the prosecution of its parts, bringing them all under one roof is no longer possible. A city is after all not too big to permit contact among men of different aptitudes and appetites. All this is correct. Extreme statements have only the value of identifying components in a complex. And yet, if cross fertilization is a desideratum, the machinery to achieve it is an object sedulously to be cultivated. The plea is to provide

[27] A. N. Whitehead, *Science and the Modern World*, New York, 1925, p. 275.

for music a richer life, to be lived intimately with fellow expressions of the spirit.

The point of my argument is this. Music is one of the arts, unlike the graphic and industrial arts, which has not found its way into museums, first because of value and also as of right. But that is just what it should do. Pieces, novel as well as old, in order to become familiar should be often repeated. The other arts are accorded this opportunity already. Music alone is denied it except in an awkward and commercialized way. Finding a legitimate home for music in museums may aid in changing an unsatisfactory form of life. At the same time the public would gain a proper place for hearing. Dignity would then come to this profession, from the beginning of a career to the arrival at fruition. And the public would own, as it does in the graphic arts, the right to become familiar with this unique, the only auditory, form of expression among the arts.

III. ARTISTS AND SCIENTISTS

In turning from art and science to scientists and artists the content of this discussion changes radically. The shift is from objective analysis of natural objects, from rational schemes, from kinship of interests, from types of expression, to the psychology of personality. Artists and scientists are commonly credited with being wholly different kinds of persons, poles apart in behavior, so different, indeed, as to be mutually ununderstandable. History and tradition have contributed to this misunderstanding. The conventional characteristics of scientists are given as Faustian—unapproachable, profound, fearsome, solitary; those of artists as gay, light-hearted, not learned, but quick-witted and companionable. What scientists do is usually vague, and their results far from understandable, certainly far from being widely understood. The world is content that they should live laborious days. For their persons, it has had no deep concern.

This difference so expressed may be greater than one may be disposed to admit, but the kernel of the statement is none the less accurate. If the circumstances of the lives of scientists were ex-

amined, the superior, not to limit these remarks to, the great ones
the most impressive quality to be disclosed would be high serious
ness, scrupulous honesty, industry and eagerness. Nor, as a matte
of fact do artists correspond to popular conceptions. Leonardo
Michelangelo, Goethe, Beethoven, Brahms, Wordsworth, Tenny-
son, Cézanne—these were neither rough nor irresponsible men
Cellinis are not difficult to find; but then, not all artists, nor al
scientists either, are cut from the same pattern. Neither is what i
caricature he is painted. Science has in fact its Lewis Carrolls.

Times change. In the tightening of the procedures of living,
all walks of life have become more tense. We live as if something were about to happen. So much has, no wish is needed to
be father of the thought. The theater in the high sense has become respectable as all big business has now come to be.

Mr. Fry [28] translates these vague reflections into more concrete
terms when he writes that:

. . . there is also an art which has withdrawn itself from the dream,
which is concerned with reality, an art therefore which is pre-eminently
objective and dis-interested, and which therefore proceeds in the opposite direction from the other kind of art. If you will admit this, the
most interesting problems suggest themselves for solution. What is the
psychological meaning of this emotion about forms, (which I will call
the passion for pure beauty), and what is its relation to the desire for
truth which is the only other disinterested passion we know of—what,
if any, are their relations to the libido and the ego?

This is, in short, a matter of psychological interest. What goes on
in the minds of artists and scientists would, if the facts were fully
known, disclose likenesses and unlikenesses of importance.

The problem is simple and concrete: How do artists come by
ideas; how do they decide what to paint or what to fashion? [29]

The usual answer given by painters and musicians (the situation is more satisfactory with poets) is that the way of their work
is by inspiration, or, as it is sometimes also called, by intuition.

[28] Roger Fry, "The Artist and Psychoanalysis," *Hogarth Essays,* New
York, 1928, p. 300.

[29] Further aspects of this problem are
discussed in the essay "The Influence of
Modern Science on Painting and Sculpture," p. 42.

The great idea is believed to enter the mind, to lie dormant, to burst forth in a moment of inspiration and then is ready to be transferred to canvas, or clay, or sound. That was Shelley's view:

Poetry is not like reasoning, a power to be exerted according to the determination of the will. A man cannot say, "I will compose poetry." The greatest poet even cannot say it; for the mind in creation is as a fading coal, which some invisible influence, like an inconstant wind, awakens to transitory brightness; this power arises from within, like the colour of a flower which fades and changes as it is developed, and the conscious portions of our natures are unprophetic either of its approach or its departure. Could this influence be durable in its original purity and force, it is impossible to predict the greatness of the result; but when composition begins, inspiration is already on the decline, and the most glorious poetry that has ever been communicated to the world is probably a feeble shadow of the original conceptions of the poet. I appeal to the greatest poets of the present day, whether it is not an error to assert that the finest passages of poetry are produced by labour and study. The toil and the delay recommended by critics can be justly interpreted to mean no more than a careful observation of the inspired moments, and an artificial connexion of the spaces between their suggestions by the intertexture of conventional expressions; a necessity only imposed by the limitedness of the poetical faculty itself; for Milton conceived the Paradise Lost as a whole before he executed it in portions. We have his own authority also for the muse having "dictated" to him the "unpremeditated song." And let this be an answer to those who would allege the fifty-six various readings of the first line of the Orlando Furioso. Compositions so produced are to poetry what mosaic is to painting. This instinct and intuition of the poetical faculty is still more observable in the plastic and pictorial arts; a great statue or picture grows under the power of the artist as a child in the mother's womb; and the very mind which directs the hands in formation is incapable of accounting to itself for the origin, the gradations, or the media of the process.[30]

And Monet said a similar thing: "No one is an artist unless he carries his picture in his head before painting it, and is sure

[30] P. B. Shelley, *Essays, Letters from Abroad.* 1852, I, p. 41.

of his method and composition." [31] To credit this conception of Shelley results in too easy an acquiescence with too partial an analysis. Ferreting out, instead, the minds and the memories of artists, studying their lives and their writings will yield the conviction that a detailed analysis of the creative process will repay closer scrutiny.

There are those who are inarticulate by nature. They cannot recall the history of an idea with any degree of minuteness or vividness or detail. They can rarely relate how a statue, a poem, a painting, originated. Their very beings require utterance in a different, a more appropriately chosen, medium, whether in sculpture or painting, or music—but not in words. Words require spelling out, time. There is no sudden burst of multi-dimensional perception, the whole translated from the conceiving mind and at once exteriorized on canvas or in stone, where the finished product is perceived. An artist may be inarticulate in any other language but his own. This was the case with Beethoven. Since the sentient life of an artist is lived exclusively in figure or paint or music, he does his communicating in these media. Mathematicians and physicists are often afflicted by a like disability. To know them you must know their language. Langmuir, Eddington, and others no doubt, as well, believe that in the future, and in certain cases even now, this kind of inarticulateness may tend to further development.

When we use the atomic or molecular theories to explain phenomena in this way we assign to the atoms and molecules only those properties which seem needed to accomplish the desired result; . . .

What we really do, therefore, is to replace in our minds the actual gases which we observe and which have many properties which we do not fully understand, by a simplified model, a human abstraction, which is so designed by us that it has some of the properties of the thing we wish to displace.

There is thus a difference of degree rather than of kind between the adoption of a mechanical model and the development of a mathema-

[31] Gustave Geffroy in *Artists on Art*, edited by R. Goldwater and M. Treves, New York, 1945, p. 313.

tical theory such as Euclidean geometry. When the mathematical physicist develops an abstract theory of actual phenomena, for example, Hamilton's equations to summarize the laws of mechanics, he is in reality constructing a mathematical model. . . .

Within recent years, especially in the development of the relativity and quantum theories, physicists have been making increasing use of mathematical forms of expression, and have been giving less attention to the development of mechanical models. The older generation of physicists and chemists and those among the younger men who are less skilled in the use of mathematics are inclined to believe that this is only a temporary stage and that ultimately we must be able to form a concrete picture or model of the atom, that is, to get a picture of what the atom is really like. It seems to be felt that a mechanical model whose functioning can be understood without the aid of mathematics, even if it only gives the qualitative representation of the phenomena in question, can represent the truth in some higher sense than a mathematical theory whose symbols perhaps can be understood only by a mathematician.

There is, I believe, no adequate justification for this attitude. Mechanical models are necessarily very much restricted in scope. The relationships of their parts are limited to those that are already known in mechanics (or in electricity or magnetism). Mathematical relationships are far more flexible; practically any conceivable quantitative or qualitative relationship can be expressed if desired in mathematical form. We have no guarantee whatever that nature is so constructed that it can be adequately described in terms of mechanical or electrical models; it is much more probable that our most fundamental relationships can only be expressed mathematically, if at all.[32]

But I venture to believe that the last word concerning mathematics versus models as methods of expression has not yet been uttered. Very likely the time has come when a bad or inadequate model will no longer pass current; but the world is tridimensional and just the sort of place which lends itself to interpretation by models. The new demand must obviously be for models that "work."

But to return to artists and their methods. What is found on

[32] I. Langmuir, "Modern Concepts in Physics and Their Relation to Chemistry," *Science*, 1929, LXX, p. 390.

paper, on canvas, or in clay, came there by no swift isolated flash—while shaving, or in the morning bath. Artists, like other people, during long lives have intricate experiences. Some are learned, and all presumably have memories. In the right mood, moved by passion, strong imagination and energy, urged on by the need for expression and, for communicating visions they discourse in their own accustomed form. Maritain believes, ". . . these sensations impinge upon consciousness only after refraction through an inward atmosphere of memories and emotions, and are besides incessantly varying, in a flux wherein all things lose their shape and continually intermingle; . . ." [33]

How the receiving mind has become the repository from which, when the occasion is ripe, experience is drawn, has been shown with extraordinary lucidity by Professor Lowes.[34] Scarcely a reference in *Kubla Khan*, but its source was traced; all emerged from the retentive storehouse of Coleridge's memory. It is unnecessary, however, to rely on a critic's analysis for the truth of the origin of the events in Coleridge's case. By good chance, Coleridge himself has circumstantially recorded the method of his thought, which, by his own beautiful induction, Professor Lowes has brought to light.

The origin of a work of art appears, in point of fact, very often to have a more intricate history. It is rarely born in the twinkling of an eye. Artists, like other sensitive people cannot avoid storing their minds. The effort that Milton made to acquire his poetical apparatus is well known. It is surely no accident that poets from Horace to Sydney, from Shelley and Wordsworth and from Goethe and Schiller to Baudelaire and Browning and in our own day to Woodberry and Eliot, all have been deeply concerned with the content and meaning and function of their art. For them poetry was not a chance occupation but, on the contrary, a high service. Nor was sculpture for Michelangelo, or Donatello, or Rodin, nor painting for Leonardo or Delacroix or Cézanne, a light concern, nor music for Handel and Beethoven and Brahms. They were all in a very literal sense, dedicated men.

---

[33] J. Maritain, *op. cit.*, p. 149.   [34] J. L. Lowes, *The Road to Xanadu*, Boston and New York, 1927.

That the minds of artists are, in Pasteur's phrase, prepared minds is wholly credible and an almost inescapable conclusion.

That superior organization of his experiences and perceptions that is effected by a genius is certainly for the most part unconscious. Numberless experiences, extending over several years, are gradually coordinated in the unconscious mind of the artist, and the total synthetic whole finds expression, it may be, on some particular occasion. Even with poetry, which often professes to have its origin in some particular occasion, the poem is never the effect of the particular occasion acting on some kind of *tabula rasa*. The experience of the particular occasion finds its place within a context, although the impact of the experience may have been necessary to bring this context to the surface. A genius may be defined as a man who is exceptionally rich in recoverable contexts. But the formation of these contexts is, for the most part, an unconscious process. A metaphor "occurs" to the poet. A musical phrase "suggests" another. And the irresistible uprising of powerful and extensive contexts may quite well induce an almost trance-like condition. To this extent not only great artists, but great philosophers and men of science, have been unconscious geniuses. Many mathematicians have been subject to trance-like conditions and, on this ground alone, there is no reason to suppose that Beethoven was more unconscious than Newton. And can we suppose that the philosopher constantly maintains in his daily life the vision of the universe that comes to him in his moments of finest insight? If we add to these considerations the possibility that Beethoven's states of illumination were not expressible in language at all, and certainly not by him, we are left with no evidence that he was an unconscious genius in any extraordinary degree.[35]

What is less evident is the extent to which actual content and arrangement to be observed in a completed work is accidental. In all probability, very little. Artists resemble the rest of mankind, especially imaginative, energetic mankind, in choosing characteristic interests peculiar to themselves. This is the fortunate circumstance which accounts for distinctiveness. What directs an interest; how closely it is determined by one's own world; what its origins are in race or family; how, by the occurrences of a lifetime a man is what he has become—a man of affairs, a scientist, a poet,

[35] J. W. N. Sullivan, *op. cit.*, pp. 130-31.

a sculptor; how it happens to be landscape,[36] the sea, animals, men, their surface, their eyes, their muscles, or still life; how an interest in atmosphere, light, line, form, or balance, Fifth Avenue, the Jungle, or Arabs, reality or symbols, may not be known, though often it can be, by patiently following the methods of search exemplified by Professor Lowes in the case of Coleridge.

The mind is stored—we say it has its "bent." Having its bent, it is precisely in the direction of that bent that it grows in wealth of knowledge and experience. This is the domain in which it exercises its selective, its critical faculties. Among the best authenticated of our experiences is a knowledge of how many factors are considered in creating a work of art, how difficult it is to satisfy a meticulous taste. It is a rare artist who erases no word, who modifies no stroke, who changes no color. We know the efforts of Monet with the haystack and the water lilies, of Cézanne with apples, of Hemingway with seventy endings! The literature of criticism exhibits many a dissertation on variant renderings. The question is not, "Does a work of art grow?" It is, rather, "How much and how often is a work of art transformed before it reaches completion?"

These reflections do not mean there is no element of chance in creation. If a work is fixed by its own contemporary scene,[37]

---

[36] "Painting is a science, and should be pursued as an inquiry into the laws of nature. Why, then, may not landscape be considered as a branch of natural philosophy, of which pictures are but experiments?" John Constable in *Artists on Art*, edited by R. Goldwater and M. Treves, New York, 1945, p. 273.

[37] In the matter of the influence of time and place I can add nothing to Maritain's statement and to one by André Gide, quoted by Maritain.

"Thus, for instance, Art as such is superior to time and place, it transcends, like the intelligence, every limitation of nationality, and finds its measure in the infinite amplitude of Beauty alone. Like Science, Philosophy, Civilization, by its very nature and by its very object it is universal. But Art has not its home in an angelic intelligence, it is subjectivised in a soul which is the substantial form of a living body; and this substantial form, by its natural need of learning and of perfecting itself by degrees and with difficulty, turns the animal it inhabits into an animal by nature political. In this way Art is fundamentally dependent on all that city and race, spiritual tradition and history bring to the body and the intelligence of mankind. By reason of its subject and of its roots it is of a par-

by the inheritance of its author, by his own life's history, what can be meant by "inspiration" and what by "intuition"? Are these essential functions? Do they serve critical ends? These are troublesome questions, and "intuition" is an especially troublesome word. It has meant different things to different men, to Croce, to Bergson, and to James. It is trying, as well as difficult, to disentangle precisely what each critic desires us to understand by his use of these terms.

A word is necessary nevertheless to denote the process that must now be described. The word "intuition" is chosen to serve this purpose and a definition for that word consistent with the usage of common sense. "Intuition," then, is the function by which, as the result of experience, usually extensive and often profound, one knows, with swiftness, what inference must be drawn in an argument or what action must be taken in a difficult situation. The phrase "experience usually extensive and often profound," is central to this problem. Antecedent, relative experience, though it is not necessary to be conscious of its possession, makes it possible in argument or in situation to arrive at a conclusion far in advance of another person, either of one inexperienced or of one not previously interested in a related problem having the current texture. Decision is quickly achieved. With surprising speed the thought perhaps of years is telescoped into an instant. To arrive at the same point, if it were possible at all, would engross laboriously the energy and the time of other men. Having lived long with a problem there is no need now, painfully and time-consumingly to rehearse the logical and successive steps. Intuition is speed made possible by experience. It need be no more. Whether without experience, a comparable rapid insight is pos-

ticular age and of a particular country." (J. Maritain, *op. cit.*, pp. 111-12.)

André Gide writes admirably: "By nationalising itself a literature takes its place and finds its significance in the concert of humanity. . . . What more Spanish than Cervantes? more English than Shakespeare? more Italian than Dante? more French than Voltaire or Montaigne, than Descartes or Pascal? what more Russian than Dostoïewsky? and what more universally human than these writers?" ("Réflexions sur l'Allemagne," *Nouvelle Revue française*, June 1, 1919.) Maritain, *op. cit.*, p. 112.

sible, cannot be known with certainty. It must be rare. This is but another way of regarding intuitions as conditioned by experience and adding that having taken thought before, thought can take place more quickly now.

Now this is the faculty which many men possess, both artists and scientists. Through it they become aware that several factors, A and B and C which had been troublesome and had long remained refractory, suddenly fall into a shape which is recognized now as being satisfactory. "Tension" is released. Why these factors A and B and C persisted in remaining refractory has so far escaped analysis. The mechanism is still a "mystery." The final act but the final act only, of the process may be designated "inspiration." When it bursts it creates a commotion. That is the moment when Archimedes jumps from his bath, runs into the street and shouts.

The mechanism of this process itself remains unanalyzed. The function is obviously not one of the conscious reason. Indeed, the conscious reason cannot force it into activity. Only this much can be said with certainty: Painful preparation by the conscious mind prepares the way for extra-conscious activity. And one other factor seems to be a condition: the unconscious mind requires peace and leisure from the importunities of conscious interference to pursue its devices in its own way. Though little is known, inquiry into the nature of this mechanism has nevertheless a long history. Having arrived at this point a notable treatise by G. B. Dibblee came by good chance into my hands. This is a painstaking study of which these reflections are confirmatory. Dibblee speaks of two forms: simple or immediate intuition, "the clever guessing founded on native shrewdness, often and especially attributed to women," for which no preparation is required, this being the same form which philosophers import "into their systems in order to provide for the elementary sensations of space-time"; [38] though this simple function is not, on further reflection, so very simple, and advanced intuition, which denotes the complex process I have been describ-

[38] *Instinct and Intuition*, London, 1929, p. 96.

ing, in which attention, perception, memory, and extra-conscious ratiocination are involved.[39]

If this is the mechanism it seems strange that we are so little aware that it is going on in our "minds." But aware of it or not, we rely upon it nevertheless. Wise men usually postpone their answers. We distrust the conscious reason of today, believing the immediate state of consciousness to be a lens which focuses the mind on a small area only of a complex content and arrangement of fact, present in the mind, all the elements of which need to be but have not yet been canvassed, and to play their role in a final result. We go still further when we distrust it even tomorrow. Many of us wait deliberately until we are assured the answer

---

[39] The following extracts can scarcely represent the learning and the care with which Mr. Dibblee has written his book. I can do no better, though, than to direct the reader's attention to the work itself: "Advanced intuition is more complicated in its operation than immediate or primary intuition, but it is equally simple in its result. It comes into consciousness with the effect of unexpected illumination, because it emerges from extra-conscious conditions into the scope and purview of a mind whose conscious side is under the inflexible impression that all its operations have been conscious. A simple mind may have experiences of this kind and simple minds may have them so often that they place in them a mistaken confidence and take easily to guessing, to reliance on 'hunches,' or on superstitions. A trained mind yields to the disclosures of intuition less easily and only after greater previous effort by the reason. Where resistance to intuitive suggestion becomes frequent in a trained mind, or specially prolonged as no doubt occurred in the case of Descartes, the simplicity and suddenness of a satisfactory solution of personal problems and particularly of acute dilemmas may easily have an explosive effect." (Dibblee, *op. cit.*, p. 98.)

"Comparing intuition with thought, the former will probably resemble the latter, while exhibiting less of the synthetic or analytic processes of thought, which are naturally enhanced by the greater opportunities offered in consciousness. The fact that chiefly guides us through the labyrinth of the study of intuition is that it is a process not set in motion by the will, but only engendered, if at all, by roundabout methods and continuous application of effort. Intuitive thought would most probably resemble that kind of passive thought described by Jung, which is not pure association. It is important to retain a firm hold on the reality that intuition is an extra-conscious process, of which we positively and directly know nothing at all. The study of ordinary behaviour gives us no clue to it and inspection or introspection very little. We hardly even know that it is mental. Its operation, so far as we can observe it, makes one think of a ferret going into a hole in the side of a hill and coming out some way off dragging a rabbit. To follow its hidden operation we have nothing to guide us except inference, for which there is slender material." (*Ibid.*, p. 113.)

we have been seeking neglects none of the facts. I have questioned many individuals and some artists on their experience. The answer is usually brief, negative, uninforming, and lacking in illuminating detail. Not only are most men unaware of their personal experience; they are all but unaware of the influence of time and place on themselves. They escape knowing they are children of their country and of their age.

Eckermann reports a conversation in which Goethe said: "You have asked me what idea I have tried to embody in my Faust. As if I knew or could tell myself! 'From heaven, across the world, down into hell'—there is an explanation if you must have one; but that is not the idea, it is the march of the action. . . ." [40] But all this is not surprising. This is a new form of inquiry—this exploration of mental events undertaken in the effort to understand how the mind works.

We know now that answers exist. But we know also that skill and further study of the mechanism of consciousness are necessary to bring the facts to the surface and so to systematic expression. Freud has given much help here. Ideas are not created full-blown, but only after long gestation. Artists often do not tell their stories because they do not know them. With patience, just how and why a particular idea and the form of its representation was born can be discovered. Memory may be blocked. Often, owing to preoccupation with other more familiar media of expression, words as descriptive symbols have fallen into disuse. Sullivan's description of Beethoven's case is admirable. But this situation is not peculiar to artists. The same phenomenon is to be observed in scientists. During a demonstration, two of them halted in an explanation of their work, for no other reason than because they found themselves incapable of putting their ideas into words. *Their* language was mathematics. Mathematical symbols were completely natural to them and native, but not translatable, and certainly not into the idiom of common speech.

And so artists are set down as intuitive over against scientists

[40] J. P. Eckermann, *Gespräche mit Goethe*, Leipzig, 1909, Part iii, May 6, 1827.

who are to be accepted as dull and laboring. The legend of Archimedes illustrates two points. First that scientists are capable of drama and second that a discovery is a longer drawn-out process than it appears to be. His problem had lain in his mind a long time, troublesome but unresolved. It was only the solution which dawned upon him suddenly—the solution—not the problem: the problem had been an old and tantalizing companion. There are other similar anecdotes. Their solutions have all taken the same way, intuitions—though the nucleus of their thought had been slowly maturing. Harvey, in describing his discovery that the blood in animals circulates, confessed: "I frequently and seriously bethought me, and long revolved in my mind. . . ." Ultimately he was able to set the facts in order: "I began to think whether there might not be a motion, as it were, in a circle." The crux of the matter is that an unworkable machine, an uncomposed picture, an illogical argument, after reflection and trial and error, comes finally into successful operation. Picture and machine, conceived not suddenly, but after long labor, after passing through the mysterious process called "intuition," were fashioned. Mr. Dibblee gives further instances in the case of Sir William Hamilton's discovery of quaternions and the mathematical solution of a problem by M. Henri Poincaré. Poincaré says in his *Science and Method:* "Demonstration is carried on by logic, but discovery is a matter of intuition. The faculty which makes us see is intuition." [41] It is, in a way, an unfortunate word, this word intuition, which means too often, and very incorrectly, only the end of a complicated process. In the light of these reflections, what is remarkable is how these functions of intuition and inspiration came to be so closely associated with artists. The operation of the mind in both orders of men seems to be closely related. But that limits its use too narrowly. This is not a function confined to classes of persons; it operates universally.

This description of artists and scientists has proceeded, so far,

[41] For other instances see Dibblee, *op. cit.*, p. 99. G. Wallas, in *The Art of Thought* (New York, 1926), mentions that "A. R. Wallace, for instance, hit upon the theory of evolution by natural selection in his berth during an attack of malarial fever at sea" (p. 87).

as if complete identity between them were being suggested. And yet this is far from the fact. It is apparent, discounting minor and secondary characteristics, which have become exaggerated and which one can readily afford to neglect, that a gulf separates them. They are both possessed, no doubt, of the four usual functions of the mind—instinct and intuition, care for fact and concern with feeling. The importance of the function of making mental images should be thoroughly examined. This was a subject in which Galton was much interested and about which, as James shows in his long quotation (from Galton), Galton made searching inquiries:

. . . scientific men, as a class, have feeble powers of visual representation. There is no doubt whatever on the latter point, however it may be accounted for. My own conclusion is that an over-ready perception of sharp mental pictures is antagonistic to the acquirement of habits of highly-generalized and abstract thought, especially when the steps of reasoning are carried on by words as symbols, and that if the faculty of seeing pictures was ever possessed by men who think hard, it is very apt to be lost by disuse. The highest minds are probably those in which it is not lost, but subordinated, and is ready for use on suitable occasions. I am, however, bound to say that the missing faculty seems to be replaced so serviceably by other modes of conception, chiefly, I believe, connected with the incipient motor sense, not of the eye balls only but of the muscles generally, that *men who declare themselves entirely deficient in the power of seeing mental pictures can nevertheless give lifelike descriptions* of what they have seen, and can otherwise express themselves as if they were gifted with a vivid visual imagination. *They can also become painters of the rank of Royal Academicians.*[42]

James adds in a footnote:

I am myself a good draftsman, and have a very lively interest in pictures, statues, architecture and decoration, and a keen sensibility to artistic effects. But I am an extremely poor visualizer, and find myself often unable to reproduce in my mind's eye pictures which I have most carefully examined.

[42] F. Galton, *Inquiries into Human Faculty*, quoted by W. James, in *The Principles of Psychology*, New York, 1899, II, 53.

Possessing the ability to make metaphors in an exuberant degree was, in Russell's view, Bergson's undoing.[43] Here I think is room for a great deal more investigation. That claim of Galton's in italics deserves very close scrutiny.

It will turn out, I think, that the different objectives to which men dedicate themselves are not accidents, but determined. The degree to which genetic substrates, not by any means accidents, decide these matters for us, was all but unsuspected a short while ago. Hormones, male and female, also play their roles. They occur in no fixed amounts, sex by sex. The fact is important that they exist. The amounts can run parallel to psychological characteristics —though for that there is now no evidence. These are no doubt not the only determining factors. It is not a far stretch to suppose, however, that if you are *so* endowed, one form of expression is native to you; if otherwise, another. You are, in ways Gilbert did not guess, *born* to your politics—and maybe also to your psychology. But this accident in genetics, if it is an accident, decides your natural form of expression and so decides which language is your medium and so finally how you are to speak. In short, you are all of a piece, ultraviolet or infrared. *Mann spricht wie einem der Schnabel gewachsen ist.* Some use words, some use images in paint or stone, some use logic with symbols. Very few of us are confined to one of these media only. It is in these terms we become artists, scientists, or mathematicians.

Delacroix's conception may easily be an error:

The scholars do nothing, after all, but find in nature what is there. The personality of the scholar is missing in his work; he is quite different from the artist. It is the seal stamped on a work which makes it a work of art, of invention. The scholar discovers the elements of things . . . and the artist composes, invents an entity, creates, he strikes men's imaginations with the spectacle of his creatures and in a manner of his own. He sums up, he makes clear to the ordinary man who sees and feels only vaguely in the presence of nature, the sensations which things arouse in us.[44]

[43] Bertrand Russell, *A History of Western Philosophy*, New York, 1945.

[44] *Journal de Eugène Delacroix*, 4th ed.; Paris, 1926, II, 431.

Delacroix thinks that "The scholar discovers the elements of things . . . and the artist composes." This is a superficial view. Neither discovers elements; neither composes. Or, it may be better to say, both discover elements and both compose. At first glance, this view seems to do violence especially to scholars, to scientists. But what they do, really, is to try to convince themselves, and us, that the picture of the world, big or little, they form, is correct. And they do it by pulling it apart to see how it functions. That is what artists do, too, though in a different area of interest.[45] Sometimes, especially formerly when scientists did this also, they were content not to probe beneath the surface but to describe simply what that surface presented to them. A very few artists delved deeper—Leonardo and especially Michelangelo. And the meaning of this—initiation of scientific advancement by artists has formed material for a pretty controversy.[46]

But there is another problem. The methods of the earliest Greek philosophers were conditioned, quite obviously, by their time. Time was of two natures; it was time in relation to the evolution of the discussion—this was young, the discipline was young; it was a time also at which proper analytical tools were not available, mathematics and an understanding of the use of experiment. Cast in one mold, endowment leads some men in one direction, cast in another, elsewhere.

How curious we have been about the two poles appears in the reflections of Helmholtz:

On the other hand an artist or a theologian will perhaps find the natural philosopher too much inclined to mechanical and material explanations, which seem to them commonplace, and chilling to their feeling and enthusiasm. Nor will the scholar or the historian, who have some common ground with the theologian and the jurist, fare better with the natural philosopher. They will find him shockingly indifferent to literary treasures, perhaps even more indifferent than he ought to be to the history of his own science. In short, there is no denying that,

[45] In the case of vision I have analyzed this in the essay "The Influence of Modern Science on Painting and Sculpture," p. 42.

[46] William M. Ivins, Jr. Unpublished essay on Vesalius.

while the moral sciences deal directly with the nearest and dearest interests of the human mind, and with the institutions it has brought into being, the natural sciences are concerned with dead, indifferent matter, obviously indispensable for the sake of its practical utility, but apparently without any immediate bearing on the cultivation of the intellect.[47]

These summaries by Delacroix and by Helmholtz have this great value. They are descriptions employed in the most intelligent contemporary vein. But that language, for this purpose, was used, I think, for the last time. Afterwards, the idiom changed. Now we have all become scientists. We have a firmer grasp of the materials with which we deal—the psychological materials. Because of their diverse characteristics, and because in exhibiting them they demonstrate the differences under discussion, the fact remains that in the processes of their minds a certain identity is revealed, the process of "intuition." In the exercise of this function as a function there appears to be nothing essentially different between scientists and artists. Both exhibit an interest in nature and its processes, sensibility, energy, robust intelligence, the accumulation of experience, and, basic to everything else, the need to express, to convey, to teach, the need of a stimulus, an audience, though the most discriminating audience—for the most critical, because, as creators they are necessarily uniquely intelligent—is themselves.

That processes in the mind function in one and the same way in individuals apparently so diverse as poets and chemists would be difficult to test had not nature itself performed the experiment. At rare and long intervals, a man appears, who manages to embrace the requisite wide range of capabilities. Goethe was at home in poetry, in statecraft, and in science, giving himself with apparent and equal ease now to one, now to another.[48] And such a man also was Leonardo—mathematician, experimenter, inquirer, anatomist, painter, sculptor, architect, inventor, as his excursions into aeronautics demonstrate. He did far more than succeed in painting. A contrast in practice between the arts and in science can be

[47] H. Helmholtz, *op. cit.*, pp. 9-10.
[48] It is not in the current fashion to seek examples in Germany but I take comfort in my choice from H. W. Nevinson whose sturdy British bias is a stout defense.

set up. The contrast deals with the proceeds of these two forms
of activity—works of art on the one hand and the laws of nature
on the other. Subject to changes in taste or style or mores, works
of art are collected—for a variety of reasons, good and bad. But
once scientific conceptions or laws of nature are abandoned or
superseded only historians collect them, in histories of philosophy,
or as pieces of evidence to demonstrate how human intelligence
developed.

IV. AESTHETICS

A discussion of aesthetics cannot fall within the limits of this
essay. The subject itself is too multifarious—Bosanquet has required some 469 pages into which to compress merely its history.
Questions such as the fitness of objects for artistic representation;
whether and which objects are beautiful, questions concerning
concepts of beauty; as well as a definition of beauty, together with
the correlated problem of ugliness—all these are matters which
must reluctantly be passed by again.[49] And so also that other issue
which deals with the eternal fitness of things: with the unchanging
endurance of archetypes, presumably forever valid and valuable
and set apart from the hazard of caprice in judgment. Here belongs the quicksand called "taste"—taste, the evanescent butter-
fly which gains its power by securing its transient sanction from
the practices and the temper of its own time and, more heedless
still, affects an air of superiority which does not hesitate to disdain
the practices and the artistic preferences of our forebears—the
assertion of superiority being the stronger the nearer their time is
to ours.

Finally, there is the physiological study of aesthetics, a topic
Vernon Lee elucidated so well. Her's was an attempt to establish
stability of taste by relating the satisfaction of an experience to the
physiological pattern of the human organism. If a constant relation between an organism and works of art could be achieved,
much, perhaps everything, would be gained for arriving at canons
of taste and of judgment. That would do away with vagary, with

[49] See page 165.

irritability, with insecurity. For the moment it seems that change, rather than changelessness, is more agreeable and would be inescapable anyway, provided "expression" rather than "appreciation" is accepted as significant in the enterprise of this form of communication. The change from expression to appreciation is not recent, but receives more support apparently, with time. An account of the process of creation, the physiological process which has already been discussed, and other matters involving skill in technical execution—all are needed. And so also the question of the significance of audiences. These are all, for the most part, subjects having to do with the environment of art, the *milieu exterieur* in which the life of art moves and has its being. They do not involve its core or its meaning. But so much requires saying, nevertheless, in anticipation of an antithesis I wish presently to consider.

One aspect of all these issues in aesthetics should be singled out for comment. It concerns what has become a province of philosophical discussion. There was defined earlier, in discussing the meaning of science, that indispensable phase of it which insists upon making some kind of general statement, the simpler the better, about the masses of phenomena which in its various divisions science passes in review. Unless at the end of its enterprises, such statements, the laws of nature, were seen to issue, scientists would confess a sense of futility. A general statement is the end of the scientific process. General statements, my teacher, Professor George E. Woodberry, following a long tradition in literary criticism, taught, are an ineradicable need, characteristic of and native in the soul of man. That these should be the end and aim of scientific activity is generally understood. They express the passion—perhaps innate—for order. In the aesthetic effort there is, no doubt, an attempt, similar to that in science, to discover in artistic adventures comparable unifying principles. Works of art and the need to create them are among the indispensable, indeed the inescapable enterprises of mankind. What wonder that, at the dawn of critical literature, in the *Poetics,* Aristotle should have been occupied with an inductive study to find the underlying conditions of poetic pleasure.[50] One must be profoundly sympathetic to this urgency, felt by men in general and by philosophers in particular in their attempt to capture the significance of "beauty" and to attain as profound an insight as may be into the "meaning" of art. In any case aesthetics has a function here, no matter how peripheral it is to the central performance.

I have arrived at the antithesis to which I referred. It is that aesthetics does not occupy an integral part, performs no operational function, to use Professor Bridgman's phrase, in the practice of art. Aesthetics lies outside the "practice" of art as law cannot be said to lie outside the "practice" of science. If scientific practice, including the formulation of laws, valid irrespective of time and locality, constitutes the method of science, artistic practice is pre-eminently an individual experience, subject to change *with* time and place. This is perhaps not an overstatement, for aesthetics is an exclusively intellectual appraisal in a sphere which is pre-eminently and dominantly, sentient expression. Nor is it certain that, as does critical philosophy in science, aesthetic speculation influences artistic practice. And this is a consequence of the fact that the emotional experience, the feeling function, in its expression, which is art, is personal and is precious just because its value consists precisely in its discreteness, its separateness, its particularity. In science, law is integral, the inherent culmination of its process; in art, philosophy is a spectator, viewing, appraising, applauding perhaps, measuring the passing show. How aesthetics, because it is no part of its nature but is an intellectual superstructure, may be regarded as outside art, as law cannot be regarded as outside science, may now in this context be clear.

Art exists, then, as an interest in a special aspect of things in nature and in its emotional statements. This aspect it portrays and interprets, and makes us understand and appreciate nature in the degree to which artists penetrate into the essence of its meaning or significance. The process or the technique employed to make that interest manifest, is the private affair of the guild of artists.

---

[50] This form of expression may be retained, although B. Russell says induction was no part of the Greek genius.

The common man is concerned with the product—not with the mechanics nor with the process.

In science, by the same token, "the world" is not concerned, no doubt it should be, with the law of the conservation of energy, with the principles of inheritance, with the doctrine of the cellular structure of living things. Concretely, the world rejoices in the use of railways, electric light, radio-telegraphy, and airplanes, caring little for the essential thought, or for the technique or the varieties of skill which have entered into their manufacture.[51] And yet the actual practitioners in science are not without concern for skill in technical accomplishment. Just as sculptors care for the surface of marble, painters for the texture of a canvas, and poets for the sound and rhythm of words, so scientists speak of "elegance" in the quality of an argument, proof, or demonstration, the possession of which is rated a high accomplishment. Elegance is opposed to awkwardness, to redundancy, to indirection. A proof is elegant if it is neat, quick, simple, containing an element of surprise. Physicists and mathematicians are acutely aware of the difference between clumsiness and deftness in presentation. Nor are biologists without a sense for skillfulness in experimenting. If elegance, technical proficiency, the rules of the craft, are of outstanding, amounting often to crucial, importance in art, they are not without a place of honor in the operations of science.

The main contention remains: the "world" cares about the product, whether of artists or scientists, but about the theory of the performance the world can afford indifference. What needs repeating and emphasizing is that theory and law belong, tight-packed within science; but in art they *can* remain forever outside the consideration of artists. The extent to which an artist is guided by them, law and theory, is immensely varying—all the way from being unaware of their existence to the point when they are determining in the creation of a work of art.[52]

Although a discussion of aesthetics is here omitted there is still

[51] Irony has taken us for her own, since the success of atomic fission.

[52] Once, when theory did enter is discussed in the essay "The Influence of Modern Science on Painting and Sculpture," p. 42.

need for troubled disentangling of the question: What is individual and what general, respectively, in art and in science?

In very recent times the notion has been entertained that the audience of an artist need be only himself. In the case of many a man that has undoubtedly but happily not frequently been the case. Here is the doctrine of solipsism in an extreme form. But a short time only elapsed before critics, like T. S. Eliot, Professor Lowes, Maritain—men of very different schools of thought— came to see that this is futile and petulant, that this way is the way of chaos, that the arts thrive because they are social functions, "social" because they express not merely a way, any way, but a usual way of man in society. Art is a necessary outlet of expression for many individuals. Men of genius do not often transcend their time and place. But has their performance, for that reason, by later critics, been interpreted in terms divorced from their *own* setting? Is this the case with Blake or with Daumier? Variant, yes; but unresponsive to the contemporary scene, no. If there exist an eagerness in a man to be understood and a desire to exhibit his most profound insights and his most eloquent expression of them, the basis for communication is laid. Assembling works of art serves to demonstrate the existence of underlying widely accepted forms. Out of collections of similar experiences an aesthetics is eventually built. An aesthetics is, as a matter of fact, conceivable in no other terms. But by way of repetition whatever aesthetics may be, ultimate value in art resides in individual performance; the individual performer remains central. In science, in general statements, in law, the individual performer is often, too often, unhappily lost. Goethe proposes a view with a different slant, though this is not one of his happier insights.

The problems of science [said Goethe] are very often the problems of living. A single discovery can make a man famous and found his family fortune. It is for that reason that in the sciences there prevails this strict discipline, this conservatism, and this jealousy of the ideas of each other. In the domain of aesthetics, on the other hand, everything is much more flexible; its thoughts are more or less the congenital property of all men, in which success depends on treatment and execution, and for this reason occasions little envy. A single thought can become the basis of a hundred epigrams, and it remains only to discover which poet knew best how to develop this thought in the most effective and most beautiful fashion.

In science, treatment is of no importance; the whole effect is a matter of insight. There is therefore little that is general and subjective, for the individual manifestations of the laws of nature lie sphinxlike, stark, solid, and silent about us. Every phenomenon, the nature of which is perceived, is a discovery; and every discovery is a private possession. Let anyone touch one of these possessions and its owner, with all his passions, will be upon one.[53]

It is an odd turn that forces on words opposite meanings when the climate of theoretical opinion changes. In such passages, this phenomenon is recalled. The point is that such antitheses have engaged the minds of thoughtful men. Goethe employed a different denotation in his use of the word "aesthetics." The difference is time—an interval of a century. Words change their meaning. Goethe together with many other contemporary scientists believed in archetypes, and so took sides in the controversy on the origin of species with St. Hilaire against Cuvier. In science he thought there was "little that was general or subjective"—laws lay about like archetypes, requiring only to be picked up and so discovered.

It is usual to think of discovery as characteristic of science. A discovery, a specific discovery, can be made only once; no one can discover the laws of motion after Galilei; nor a law which describes a certain behavior of gases after Boyle; nor the doctrine of evolution after Darwin; nor combustion in the animal body after Lavoisier. A discovery is made once for all—forever afterward, though the experience is identified with the discoverer, the use of the discovery belongs to mankind. The statements which describe the experiments cease, however, to be adventures; they are laws. Experience passes from the particular to the general.

But in painting discoveries also are made. Paolo Uccello "discovered" perspective; someone (or a school) learned how to paint in the round; Leonardo analyzed the surface appearance of the body; Seurat stimulated by Helmholtz experimented with

[53] Eckermann, *op. cit.*, Dec. 30, 1923.

the representation of light; [54] Picasso or Braque discovered methods of presentation, superior, in their judgment, to visual accuracy —the assumption being that visual accuracy is neither accurate nor dignified.[55] These are all discoveries; new paths. What has recently been said of Paolo Uccello may be said of all of these. "Almost all the greatest artists . . . seem to have been much concerned with intellectual problems and yet always in the end to have changed an intellectual problem into one of sensibility." [56] It is generally believed that art affords opportunities for the display of individuality that science does not possess. A collection of the portraits of Harvey, of Shakespeare, and of Maria Lani demonstrates amply what is well known in every school where students study a model. The landscapes that *can* be painted are innumerable, yet those that have been, fall into types; background landscapes in the Italian Renaissance, the landscapes of contemporary Sweden, those of Hobbema, the landscape of Ruysdael, of Claude Lorrain, or of Watteau, the landscape of François Millet or of Cézanne. These become models which innumerable people imitate. The end is multiplicity of examples until finally the result is boredom—mass handicraft but not a "law."

In science on the contrary, advance moves from idea to idea, from proof to proof, making the history of science look as if it were determined. But progress is not consistent. Lags have existed and fruitless bypaths have been followed. In point of fact the march forward has been halting, centuries separating its steps, for reasons not always clear. From Aristotle to Pliny, from Galen to

[54] Clive Bell, *Landmarks in Nineteenth Century Painting*, New York, 1927, p. 195.

[55] "The intellect is bound to seek for articulations. In order to handle nature's continuity it has to be conceived as discontinuous; without articulation, without organization, the intellect gets no leverage. And with Cézanne, the intellect—, or to be more exact, the intellectual part of his sensual reactions—claimed its full rights. From this point of view we may regard the history of art as a perpetual attempt at reconciling the claims of the understanding with the appearances of nature as revealed to the eye at each successive period. Each new discovery in the world of visual experience tends to invalidate the constructions which had proved adequate therefore, and the spirit is bound to reconstruct its shelter, taking into account the new data." (Roger Fry, *Cézanne. A Study of His Development*, New York, 1927, p. 40.)

[56] From review in *Literary Supplement, The Times*, London, December 5, 1929.

Vesalius, from Ptolemy to Copernicus, from Mayow to Lavoisier, from Newton to Einstein, from Dalton to Rutherford, long quiescent periods intervened. Even if a sort of inexorableness were driving science on, from discovery to discovery it still remains that the next "inevitable" development is unperceived.

They, art and science, are both alike here. Progress, the next step, is hidden. Chance does no more than accommodate, favor, meet a prepared mind. The prepared mind rarely manufactures the chance without strong accidental support. There is nothing inevitable or inescapable. In the arts, although change—not necessarily advance—is possible, many influences play important, if not decisive, roles. Contrariwise art, less driven than science, is not quite free from an inner compulsion to evolve. Greek sculpture which took to perfecting its types, as Gisela Richter tried to demonstrate, makes one doubt the existence of freedom. Art is not free to follow implicit fancies. Greek naturalism was followed by the formalism of Byzantium.

No one will conclude, I hope, that identity between art and science is being asserted here, but remote similarity only. Nor will anybody infer that the emotions pursue a course, whatever it may be, parallel with that of the intellect. As these functions differ so do their expressions. But the central point is that it is not without interest, and not without surprise either, to become aware of unsuspected likenesses in their operation, and so to realize that the nature of man, so long regarded as split, is one and that with understanding its two aspects can achieve harmonious interplay.

If Nature engrosses the attention of men in moods so different as art and science, in scientists and artists she yet exhibits a surprising uniformity in the mental processes which make the effort to understand her. At the same time likeness in mental processes does not spell identity in endowment, and difference in endowment obviously compels difference in expression.

The argument in this essay was designed to show forth that between science and art there was this difference: whereas it was in the nature of science to be general, it was in the nature of art to be individual. As the analysis has proceeded, it has become evident that science is far from being without its fallible human aspect or far from being undeviatingly progressive. And art, far from being the plaything of the individual fancy, exhibits unanticipated internal rigor and consistency. Instead of being free in the sense that each individual makes his own arbitrary contribution, in art too, its supreme professors make general discoveries. These become everybody's possessions and, due to innovations, the stage is set for a next development both in the technique and in the content of expressiveness. There is value in antithesis. But antithesis unmodified by the nuances which fineness of sensibility perceives would lead not to truth but to error. Art is not science, nor is thought emotion, but they share in that which is lent to them by their common origin in the curiosity of man.

The Development of the Harveian Circulation

YOUR request, Mr. President, that I deliver this address commemorating the tercentenary of the publication of William Harvey's *Exercitatio anatomica de motu cordis et sanguinis in animalibus* gave me the liveliest pleasure and afforded me a welcome opportunity. I come to you fresh from the study of a genuinely towering intellect, inspired by the life of a great physician, full of admiration for the nature of his investigations and of the manner of his thought. I am to speak of William Harvey, an ornament to mankind.

A review of Harvey's life leaves the impression that here was a man unusually favored by fortune, one who utilized with great intelligence the rare opportunities which the contemporary world afforded. For William Harvey, in view of the discovery he was to make, was singularly fortunate in the century, and in precisely the period of that century, in which he was born; he was fortunate in his family and in the support and strength which they brought to his aid; his college was chosen for him with extraordinary prescience; he came to Padua just at the right moment; on his return to England he became associated with, and was soon elected a Fellow of, the Royal College of Physicians of London; he was chosen physician to St. Bartholomew's Hospital within seven years after attaining his degree; the coveted Lumleian lectureship in anatomy at the College became his in 1615 at the age of 37 and afforded him in the next year the opportunity of teaching for the first time that the blood in the body of animals circulates. He was fortunate, finally, in his friends, many of whom were devoted to his person; in the fame which came to him in full measure; in the great length of his life of eighty years spent in the complete enjoyment of intellectual vigor.

He was a man of rather low stature, olive complexion, of moderate portliness, if one may judge from the numerous portraits still extant, dark of hair and piercing dark of eye, quick, perhaps abrupt in his gestures, moved easily to anger, but direct, imperious, jealous of the prerogatives of his calling, as witness his St. Bartholomew's reforms,[1] but kindly withal, as his friendships with Nardi, Ent, Scarborough, and Thomas Hobbes amply show.

It is less on his life, though, than on his thought that I wish to dwell. And because there seems to be direction in his course, beginning with his entrance at Gonville and Caius College in Cambridge in 1593 when he was but 15 years of age, we do well to begin at this point. In all probability, the atmosphere of no other college could have directed his attention as this one may have done to anatomical studies. The second founder and Master, John Caius, was himself a physician, most exceptional when heads were usually churchmen. He secured for his college and for Harvey two things of importance: an interest in anatomy and a contact with Padua where he had been student and professor. Caius returned to England in about 1544. Two years later he was giving anatomical lectures and demonstrations at the hall of the barber surgeons, the first to be given in England, in which he revealed to this fraternity "the hidden jewels and precious treasures of Cl. Galenus, showing himself to be the second Linacer." He did, moreover, obtain for his college of Gonville and Caius "the grant of a charter by which the Master and Fellows were allowed to take annually the bodies of two criminals condemned to death and executed in Cambridge or its Castle free of all charges to be used for the purpose of dissection, with a view to the increase of the knowledge of medicine and to benefit the health of her Majesties lieges." Unfortunately, it is not known certainly whether this privilege was used or whether Harvey was

[1] Sir Norman Moore, *The History of
St. Bartholomew's Hospital*, London,
1918, II, 491.

exposed to that influence of which this charter was an expression. Caius, like Linacre before and many other Englishmen after him, had been attracted to the anatomical lectures at Padua, where he spent somewhat more than five years. He formed a close acquaintance with Vesalius and was indeed his fellow-lodger for eight months in the Casa degli Valli just at the time when Vesalius was busy writing his *De fabrica humani corporis*. Later, in 1543, he began a journey through the great cities of Italy in the attempt to obtain in their libraries complete and correct versions of Hippocrates and Galen. Venn [2] tells us that, of the nine volumes of manuscripts in the library of Caius College given by the Master, the majority consist of treatises written by them. Himself a Paduan, an anatomist, a disciple of Galen and Hippocrates, a student of Vesalius trained in the great Paduan tradition, this was the Master of Harvey's College. It is now known on the authority of Sir Thomas Barlow [3] and of Venn that Harvey was enrolled a minor pensioner on a scholarship. This particular scholarship was granted at the Grammar School at Canterbury, Harvey's school, to students who were intending to study anatomy and medicine, and had been established on the advice of Caius. The choice of college therefore, if deliberate, was wise; if accidental, fortunate. Caius had been dead (1573) five years when Harvey was born (1578) and twenty when he came to Cambridge (1593).

In 1598, or as Barlow thinks in 1600, with this background, Harvey at 20 entered Padua. Here he lived for four or, more probably, for two years. Padua must then have been in veritable ferment. Within the century the leaders at Padua, as Sir George Newman reminds us,[4] were an anatomist, a practitioner, a professor, and a physicist—Vesalius, Fracastorius, Fabricius, Galilei. Galilei had been there since 1592. The *aula magna* where he taught adjoined the anatomical theater. "In 1593, after Fabricius had been professor for thirty years, the Venetian authorities erected

[2] *The Works of John Caius, with a Memoir of His Life by John Venn*, Cambridge, 1912.

[3] Sir Thomas Barlow, "Harvey, The Man and the Physician," *British Medical Journal*, 1916, II, 577.

[4] *Interpreters of Nature*, London, 1927.

for him a small circular theatre which still exists, and here Harvey learned at his feet."

Of Harvey's life in Padua all too little is known. He was a member of the more select *Universitas juristarum*, and he must have attained some prominence, for he was elected *conciliarius* of the English nation. His teachers were Fabricius ab Aquapendente in anatomy, Minadous in medicine, and Casserius in surgery. He is believed to have been on terms of friendship with Fabricius, for whom throughout his life, as his two treatises show, he entertained sentiments of admiration and affection. After the negative one by Vesalius, it was Fabricius who made the one significant contribution to the knowledge of the anatomy of the organs of the circulation since Galen, fourteen centuries before. The valves of the veins had been known to Jacobus Sylvius, but his description of them had been forgotten, and they were rediscovered by Fabricius in 1574. Harvey may have learned about them directly from the Master, but Fabricius' book *De venarum ostiolis* was not published until 1603, the year after Harvey returned to England. Great seminal years these must have been, for the interests then aroused are reflected in the two treatises of Harvey that have come down to us. Beside the book on the veins, Fabricius wrote one also called *De formatione ovi et pulli* (1600).

Fabricius was followed in Padua by Casserius and Spigelius, but the great tradition was drawing to an end. With Harvey it passed to England, with Bauhin to Basel, with Bartholin to Copenhagen, with Malpighi to Bologna.

As at Cambridge, so in Padua, the attempt is baffling to reconstruct the influences which were exerted on Harvey. There were Fabricius and Galilei; there was the tolerant religious spirit of the Venetian republic, free to Protestant as well as to Catholic Europe; there was the tradition of doubt, the spirit of intellectual freedom; there was, indeed, the absorbing interest in the entire scientific Renaissance; but what would one not give for reports of the very lectures, the intimate conversations and the spirited discussions, without doubt not always pacific, which kept the town in a ferment of philosophical speculation. This is the knowledge that would give us real insight into what Harvey had stored in his mind as he turned toward England in 1602. Unfortunately, all is veiled in mystery. Galilei influenced him no doubt—see the use, for instance, that he made of arithmetic in calculating the volume output of the heart, perhaps the most striking argument employed in his proof that the blood circulates.

Between 1602, the year of his return to England and 1616 when he began to deliver the Lumleian lectures at the Royal College of Physicians, the facts of his life are known but the detail is scant. He became Doctor of Medicine at Cambridge (1602), and years later at Oxford; he married; he was appointed (1609) physician to St. Bartholomew's Hospital; he became Fellow (1607) of the Royal College of Physicians of London. But what his thought was, with whom he associated, what experiments he performed, all is obscure.

The obscurity ceases in the year 1616, the year of greatest importance in tracing the development of Harvey's thought. He was now thirty-eight years old. He had been appointed fourth Lumleian lecturer the year before (August 4, 1615), according to custom, for life. Originally, the lecturer was enjoined to lecture twice a week throughout the year, to wit Wednesdays and Fridays, at ten of the clock until eleven. He was to read for three-quarters of an hour in Latin and the other quarter in English, "wherein that shall be plainly declared for those that understand not Latin." It was his office to lecture upon the entire subject of anatomy and surgery which, for the purpose, was divided and delivered part by part, over a period of six years. Harvey was now to deliver his first course. The function was surrounded by an elaborate ceremonial. A company of great distinction was present. Although they may not have numbered above forty in all from the college, many of the curious of the town, like Evelyn, Digby, Browne, and Pepys, may have been present. The lectures were delivered in the college, which two years before had been removed from Linacre's own house in Knightrider Street, to Amen Corner at the end of Paternoster Row. It is not altogether clear whether Harvey accurately followed the traditional order, but it is certain that this first course of the visceral lectures was delivered on Tuesday, Wednesday, and Thursday, April 16, 17, and 18, 1616. A week this was of poignant interest to all those interested in the march of great events in the English-speaking world, for on the Tuesday next following, April 23, the life of William Shakespeare ended at Stratford-on-Avon, and there two days later he was laid to rest in the chancel of the parish church.

It is important to dwell with emphasis on the Lumleian lectureship, and on his lecture notes *Prelectiones anatomiae universalis,* for they mark the date of Harvey's great departure from tradition. They contain complete evidence that what subsequently came to be recognized as the Harveian circulation was already clearly defined in Harvey's mind. He delayed the publication of the results of his observation for twelve years; but in the letter of dedication to Doctor Argent, President of the Royal College of Physicians, and to his colleagues which accompanied the *Exercitatio* of 1628, he recalls what they must have known very well:

I have already and repeatedly presented you, my learned friends, with my new views of the motion and function of the heart, in my anatomical lectures; but having now for nine years and more confirmed these views by multiplied demonstrations in your presence, illustrated them by arguments, and freed them from the objections of the most learned and skilful anatomists, I at length yield to the requests, I might say entreaties, of many, and here present them for general consideration in this treatise.[5]

His book was apparently far from being a new story.

What Harvey's views actually were and how he sought to demonstrate their correctness I mean to analyze later in detail. But in order to understand them, it is necessary to understand the foundation on which he built. For Harvey was not only an original investigator but was, over and above this, a profound and learned scholar. He knew all the anatomists and the great writers of the classical world. He knew Hippocrates; Aristotle, whom he mentioned as many as fifty times in the notes alone; and Galen. He knew them all; indeed, he knew them well. They do, in fact, ill serve his reputation who undervalue them—their acumen and

[5] "An Anatomical Disquisition on the Motion of the Heart and Blood in Animals" in *The Works of William Harvey.*   Translated by Robert Willis, London, 1847, p. 5.

intelligence, the careful and logical consideration which they, the great thinkers from Aristotle to Fabricius, had devoted to solving the problems of the blood and its motion. For it was these men to whom ultimately he rose superior. The study had in point of fact gone forward in relatively few stages. Aristotle built in large measure on his predecessors and was soon followed by the very acute anatomists at Alexandria, especially by Erasistratus. After them no considerable change was introduced until the close study which Galen gave to this problem. And after him the names of three men only need be mentioned to complete the record of significant contributions before the time of Harvey; they are Vesalius, Realdus Columbus, and Fabricius.

The ancients in this connection were challenged by three great riddles: the source of animal heat, the meaning of respiration, the function of the blood.

The blood was known to be of two kinds, arterial and venous, different in color and contained, respectively, in the arteries and veins. Pulsation resulted from a force innate in the blood. All the arteries pulsated in unison and synchronously with the heart. The two bloods moved slowly to and fro, each in its channel. It must be clearly understood that slow motion was required to permit time for the exchange of substances between each blood and the tissues. To the ancients the idea that this might be accomplished rapidly was inconceivable, and remained so even in the arguments which Riolanus the Younger made against Harvey.

The function of the *venous* blood was to collect nutritive material from the intestines and to transport this by the portal vessels for further elaboration by the liver into *natural* spirits. Its onward course is a matter of first importance. On leaving the liver this blood, the venous blood, *the* blood according to Galen, divided, passing downward and upward. A small amount only, and this also is important, was diverted to what is now known as the right auricle but was then regarded merely as a dilatation of the caval system (superior and inferior *venae cavae*). It passed next through the tricuspid valve and onward to the lungs through the pulmonary artery. The smallness of the amount which reached the right ventricle and the lungs is a major conception which permitted the maintenance of the ancient system and remained to dog the reforms of Servetus, Columbus, and Caesalpinus.

The *arterial* blood also moved in a slow tidal fashion. It conveyed two things: first the pneuma, a subtle constituent of the air, which was for the function of life an essential element. The pneuma entered the blood in the lungs whence it was carried by the pulmonary veins to the left ventricle, there further to be elaborated into *vital* spirits. The second was heat which was stored in, and elaborated by, the heart itself. These two qualities, vital spirits and heat, were conveyed thence to the tissues. That portion of the arterial blood which went to the brain was further elaborated there into animal spirits, or better perhaps called psychic spirits. So refined, this substance passed along the nerves, ultimately to find its way back into the main stream by the veins. This is a Galenic account. But they were already old functions at the time of Galen, who, according to Allbutt,[6] conceived them much less clearly than had the Ionian Greeks. Heraclitus's animating fire was "something between air and flame, penetrating and vitalizing everything," something subtler than animating fire. Straton, a later member of the school of Aristotle, "held that the spirit was carried in by the semen." And so, says Allbutt, "the idea of combustion was lost."

It must be understood distinctly that the heart conveyed no propelling motion to the two bloods. It was clear that it was subject to motion; but the motion was bellows-like, a motion of sucking in, what would now be called a motion of active diastole. It was not the function of this motion to propel blood to the periphery, but to draw blood into its cavities, to churn and to agitate it as might be done in a mixing-chamber. How little motion was conceived to be conveyed to the blood, its heat and spirits, and how little desirable this motion was regarded to be, is gained from the opinion of Dr. Thomas Winston (1575-1655), professor of physic at Gresham College, who feared these (i.e., the blood, heat, and spirits) might "be broken with continuall motion."

[6] Sir T. Clifford Allbutt, "The Innate Heat." *Contributions to Medical and*   *Biological Research,* dedicated to Sir William Osler, New York, 1919, I, 219.

The motion of the blood was, as has been said, slow and tide-like. Actually, small quantities only moved, drops or the fractions of drops as Riolanus (1580-1657) supposed. In one's waking hours it moved out toward the periphery and back again to the heart during sleep. This motion was actually retained by Caesalpinus, he whom the Italians credit with the discovery of what is now called the "circulation."

The double vascular system which has been described gave rise to two divergent views, those respectively of Aristotle and of Galen. In Aristotle's scheme the heart was the center of the physiological mechanism; here arteries and veins both took their origin, and to the heart both bloods were returned, once a day, as Empedocles taught, each to its appropriate side. The parallel system resulted from the bilateral formation of the body. There were no anastomoses; [7] there was, as yet, no great elaboration of the system of the spirits. To Galen this arrangement seemed impossible; it permitted entrance from, though there could be no return of blood to, the *venae cavae* once it became trapped by the tricuspid valve. The small quantity of blood which passed through this orifice and on into the pulmonary artery could be accounted for—it served a purpose. But the major portion was believed not to enter the heart. Galen regarded the liver as the center and source of the vascular system and the originator of the blood. He took into consideration, furthermore, that the portal system led to the liver, so that three, rather than two, vascular systems met here—obviously a more important resort than the heart. These divergent views were still living issues in the first quarter of the 17th Century; physicians were divided into two camps, ranged one with Aristotle, the other with Galen. It was the famous conflict between the philosophers and the physicians in which the philosophers, gallantly led by Harvey, finally won. This controversy gives meaning to Harvey's statement in his letter to Slegel: "As Dean of the College of Paris, he was bound to see the physic of Galen kept in good repair, and to admit no novelty into the school, without the most careful winnowing." Riolanus was dean in Paris, and Paris was for the camp of Galen.

[7] Communication between two vessels.

So far the two bloods, arterial and venous, have been described as being quite different and having no method of intercommunication. In point of fact, each was thought to exhibit in slight degree characteristic properties of the other, as if we should say both contained appropriate concentrations of oxygen and carbon dioxide. Communications were, in fact, believed to exist, at the periphery, in the heart, and in the lungs. Erasistratus, because the arteries were empty after death, regarded them as containing only spirits during life. But he noticed that, when an artery was punctured, it bled; he wisely concluded that, somehow, blood passed from the veins wherein it was contained to the arteries from which it flowed, and therefore he invented anastomoses, structures which remained respectable parts of anatomy until Harvey dealt away with them. These anastomoses must not be confused with those of a later time, for in them blood flowed in two directions, like a tide. That the arteries actually contained blood was demonstrated by Galen in many experiments. In his most famous one he trapped blood between two ligatures; on being incised, it was obvious that the artery contained blood. Through the septum of the heart also, blood passed by small invisible and tortuous pores to be elaborated in the left ventricle into vital spirits. The septal passage also was Galen's suggestion. Finally, an interchange of blood in the lungs was regarded as necessary, for blood certainly passed from the *venae cavae* into the right ventricle and thence into the lungs, where the natural passed through the first stage of elaboration into vital spirits. But since the pulmonary valves prevented its return, this blood, small in amount perforce, flowed onward into the pulmonary veins, squeezed into them by the collapse of the lungs. Galen's plan came perilously near that proposed by Servetus and Columbus.

To the lungs themselves, the ancients, the moderns, and Harvey himself attributed four distinct functions. First they were presumed to aid in maintaining the tide of the blood by their rise and fall. In the second place, from the air, they *admitted* substances essential to life; while the blood brought to them by the pulmonary veins *discharged* through them fuliginous vapors, excrementitious in nature. These veins provided a possible channel because the mitral valve formed of two only, instead of three, cusps was, so Galen believed, imperfect. The blood flowed here, therefore, in two directions. But the third was the most important; it was the office of the lungs to ventilate and to cool the blood, warmed sometimes to boiling by the innate heat of the heart. Aside from these three functions, the lungs protected the heart—that most important of all the organs, the very center of life itself. Finally, the lungs shared with the heart, the coction, the elaboration of the vital spirits.

Beyond the facts of anatomy already discovered, the ancients were confronted with a number of phenomena which challenged explanation. They inferred from crude experiment that breathing was essential to life, was perhaps the source of life itself. And they knew other things. They knew, for example, that the heart tapped against the chest wall; they knew that the heart was muscular; they knew that the valves of the heart functioned; they knew that the arteries pulsated; they knew that arteries and veins were connected with the heart and that the arteries and veins contained blood different in color—truly a bewildering array of facts. One must read Galen to appreciate the excellence of the system he instituted, its internal coherence, its consideration of all these and other matters including the change from fetal to the post-embryonic circulation. Beside problems obviously connected with the circulation, they were puzzled, as I have said, by the problem of animal heat. That heat was necessary they surmised, for was it not a commonplace observation that, when alive, the body was warm, but cold when dead? A probable locus for the generation and storage of the innate heat they knew must exist. What more natural than that the heart should be selected for this purpose? Its location and vascular connections suggested its choice as the most convenient source from which to distribute heat; the heart presented the advantage, moreover, of close proximity to the lungs, where it could be cooled and tempered. Their choice was wise and has been justified by time.

Let those who never theorize beyond the facts criticize these ancient conclusions or regard their authors as ignorant or merely perverse. Was it not Galen who in his own life put blood into the arteries, saw that the heart is muscular, recognized the function of the valves, though, when convenient in debate, he conceived their closures to be imperfect; recognized the difficulty of tidal flow in the veins and right ventricle in the face of a competent tricuspid valve? He had, moreover, to see to it that spirits both natural and vital were finally conveyed to the left ventricle. And in order to perform this feat, was he not obliged to invent pores in the septum, much as Harvey in his time invented pores in the lungs and flesh—a supposition which Malpighi later established as a fact? Nor at the mention of his name should I fail to recall that we are this year celebrating another tercentenary, that, namely, of the birth of the ingenious Malpighi himself.

It is to the lasting honor of Vesalius that, on the assurance of his senses, he cured the heart of this Galenic defect of the septum and, by so doing, set the stage for a new scene. After Vesalius a new pathway from veins to arteries had, of necessity, to be found. Had Galen known the valves of the veins, knowledge of the one significant structure added after his time to the common stock, what use he would have made of them is an interesting speculation. Original and bold, he would surely have felt himself compelled to introduce them into his system. He might have failed in making the great discovery, but how many of the necessary data he had in hand! Galen himself has illuminating remarks to make on the conditions which govern discovery. He, like so many other questioners, wondered, as Dalton points out, why truth is often so long obscured by the errors of the past:

One may naturally ask [Galen inquires] how it is that men of so much intelligence could have maintained an opinion so contrary to the truth, since they must have had some plausible reason for their belief? To which I reply that they have left on record in their writings the grounds on which their belief was founded; and these grounds, though plausible, are not really sufficient. In such matters a frequent source of error is the following. Everything which comes under the cognizance of human intelligence is comprehended either through the senses or by the reason; and as there are many things of a physical nature which escape the senses, so our reason often fails to master those of a different kind. A sincere lover of the truth, therefore, should never withhold his assent from things plainly evident on account of others which are obscure, nor accept those which are doubtful for the sake of what is really known. . . .[8]

A profound saying this, circumstantially repeated by Harvey himself in the introduction to his *De generatione,* forever requiring reiteration in the pursuit of a mistress so plausible as Nature.

The contribution of Vesalius has already been mentioned. So has the rediscovery of the valves of the veins. Fabricius had, as a matter of fact, no real use for them. He was, indeed, inclined to believe that they protected the veins from rupture by impeding the tendency to a rapid downward flow of blood, a service which was performed in the arteries by their heavier coats. Fabricius, great as he was, was no Galen.

But the episode of the discovery of the pulmonary circuit requires more detailed consideration though there is reason to believe that its significance has been somewhat exaggerated. Harvey was familiar with the account Columbus gave of it in 1559 but does not mention the earlier one, rendered much more interesting on account of its theological bias, and published by Servetus in his *Christianismi restitutio* (1553). To Harvey it was scarcely more important than Galen's speculation, for he says in a parenthesis in his letter to Slegel:

. . . Riolanus uses his utmost efforts to oppose the passage of the blood into the left ventricle through the lungs, and brings it all hither through the septum, and so vaunts himself on having upset the very foundations of the Harveian circulation (although I have nowhere assumed such a basis for my doctrine; for there is a circulation in many red-blooded animals that have no lungs). . . .[9]

Nevertheless, by suggesting the pulmonary transit, contact between air and venous blood for partial purification was properly provided for. Incidentally, as Professor Curtis remarks, the Galenic defect of the imperfect mitral valve was cured. But neither Columbus nor Servetus did the Galenic system any real

[8] J. C. Dalton, *Doctrines of the Circulation,* Philadelphia, 1884, p. 74.

[9] Harvey, "Letter to Paul Marquard Slegel," *op. cit.,* p. 597.

damage. In reality they strengthened it, for both continued to maintain that *a small portion only* of the venous blood passed the tricuspid valve and moved onward to the left ventricle. The valves, by the change in direction of blood flow, became competent, but the erroneous system was unshaken. The main portion of the venous blood still remained in the *venae cavae* outside the heart and continued there its tidelike career. The new system was small gain, indeed, since by rescuing the valves from incompetence the old system was apparently more firmly intrenched and the chance of discovering *the* circulation more definitely postponed. From the Galenic point of view the great gain was that the heart was still safe from the entrance of crude venous blood. Proof, indeed the very suggestion, was still to be made that the whole blood, and not merely a small fraction of it, traversed the lungs.

Frazer dwells with much interest on the situation brought about by the writing of Servetus and Columbus, and concludes justly:

All these anatomists have been credited, at one time or another, with knowledge of the circulation, but if we turn to their accounts of the veins and liver—a very good test of their views—it is found that they were all quite innocent of any conception of the circulation. . . . In all these cases the passage through the lungs, which had been postulated by Galen, was simply adopted to supply the left heart with the material for its manufacture of "vital spirits," the perforations in the septum having lost caste with most writers.[10]

Certain it is, that the method, the temper, the character of the intellect, displayed in the writings of Harvey are in such sharp contrast to those of his forerunners as to introduce the student of his treatise into a new world. His is no longer the vague, unsatisfying recital of incompletely observed events, but the firm and thorough description of a genuinely accurate observer. I omit all mention of Caesalpinus, who, though interesting in himself, and no doubt entitled to some credit in the history of this matter, seems to have played no part in Harvey's discovery.

[10] J. Ernest Frazer, "The Harveian Lecture on The Heart before Harvey," *British Medical Journal,* 1924, I, 1083.

It is time to return to Harvey and to an analysis of his reasons for dissatisfaction with the inherited beliefs. There are, so far as they are known to me, three sources of information which suggest whence the hint came to Harvey that the blood actually circulates. According to Sir Norman Moore, the dawn of the idea is to be inferred from a note in his own *Prelectiones*, in which Harvey himself attributed to Aristotle the suggestion that led to his proof. The second, I take from the Honourable Robert Boyle:

And I remember [writes Boyle] that when I asked our famous *Harvey*, in the only Discourse I had with him, (which was but a while before he dyed) What were the things that induc'd him to think of a *Circulation of the Blood?* He answer'd me, that when he took notice that the Valves of the Veins of so many several Parts of the Body, were so Plac'd that they gave free passage to the Blood Towards the Heart, but oppos'd the passage of the Venal Blood the Contrary way: He was invited to imagine, that so Provident a Cause as Nature had not so Plac'd so many Valves without Design: and no Design seem'd more probable, than That, since the Blood could not well, because of the interposing Valves, be Sent by the Veins to the Limbs; it should be Sent through the Arteries, and Return through the Veins, whose Valves did not oppose its course that way.[11]

The third source is Harvey himself in the introduction to his book, where the reason assigned in his conversation with Boyle is, most curiously, omitted. He dwelt *first* and also longest on the error then current that the pulse and the respiration served identical ends, ". . . whether with reference to purpose or to motion, comporting themselves alike." Of this belief he disposed by showing that lungs and heart were strikingly different in structure and that the arteries never contained air. The older authors were, furthermore, in contradiction with one another on all important points. *Second*, he found it impossible to believe that the heart, arteries, and veins all beat synchronously and that the wave of the pulse passed, as Galen supposed, along the wall rather than along the fluid column. *Third*, he could not conceive why different

[11] *A Disquisition about the Final Causes of Natural Things*, London, 1688, p. 157.

functions should be assigned to the two ventricles, the left only to elaborate vital spirits. *Fourth,* he could not see why, whenever it suited the argument, anatomists declared the four great cardiac valves to be permeable, and especially the mitral valve, which was permitted to pass fuliginous vapors but not the vital spirits. *Fifth,* he was overwhelmed by the variety of functions assigned to the weak-walled pulmonary veins as against the stronger pulmonary artery, and was especially concerned about the to-and-fro motions of the blood which the systems then current postulated must take place within the lumen of its walls. *Sixth* and finally, he saw no reason for maintaining the existence of the pores of the septum, when in the first place they could not be found, and in the second, when motion through them was conceived to pass only from right to left and never in the contrary direction. To Harvey, writing before the days of Stephen Hales, this seemed an irrational position. This list of objections clearly bristles with formidable difficulties. Harvey's acumen in marshaling its items raises him at once far above the level of his contemporaries. Having given sufficient reasons for embarking upon his undertaking, one the more necessary to him because "Hieronymus Fabricius of Aquapendente, although he has accurately and learnedly delineated almost every one of the several parts of animals in a special work has left the heart alone untouched," and having stated that he had almost, like Fracastorius, resigned an understanding of this organ to God, he launched out upon his great demonstration.

The argument, continued through seventeen short chapters, begins simply enough but accumulates force until at the end it becomes overwhelming. Whereas his predecessors had assigned to the blood the sort of motion it should theoretically exhibit, Harvey proceeded differently. He studied the heart itself, not in one animal, but in animals of many species. He looked at the heart; [12] he removed it from the body; he held it in his hands. He saw that its great function was to contract; that, when doing so, it became smaller, harder, and paler; that, by doing so, it developed enough energy to expel blood. And then he noticed—

[12] Harvey, "An Anatomical Disquisition, etc.," chap. ii.

great discovery—that the apex of the heart, when in place, struck
the chest, not in diastole, as had been universally believed, but
in systole. It followed logically that if, during systole, the ventricles discharged blood, the arteries must dilate, not as a bellows
to draw in blood but like a glove into which something is forced.[18]
So perished the notion of the simultaneous contraction of heart,
arteries, and veins. A more detailed examination of the motions
of the heart showed [14] that auricles, and ventricles also, contracted
not synchronously but in succession, four motions at two times,
not four motions at four times, as Riolanus and Bauhin taught.
He found evidence for this in the phenomena of the dying heart
now so familiar, the *ultimum moriens,* and the incomplete heart-
block of asphyxia. He proved, furthermore, that the auricles
pumped blood into the ventricles. He saw, in the hen's egg, how
"a drop of blood makes its appearance which palpitates, as Aristotle had already observed." He believed that the auricles, the
last to die, were also the first to live, the *primum vivens.* To the
palpitating drop of blood we shall return. He found, in short, that
the auricles contract first,[15] send blood into the ventricles, and
that these contract in turn. To drive home the kind of motion
which he had in mind, he resorted to two illustrations: first to
firearms, in which the mechanism is a chain of successive acts—
trigger, flint and steel, spark, powder, flame, explosion, ball;
and second to deglutition, to the passage of a morsel from the
mouth through successive structures to the stomach. And in this
connection he becomes a forerunner of Laënnec by mentioning
in passing boldly and without ornament:

. . . when a horse drinks . . . the motion being accompanied with
a sound . . . ; in the same way it is with each motion of the heart,
. . . that a pulse takes place, can be heard within the chest.

In the next sentence he came to one of his important conclusions.

. . . the one action of the heart is the transmission of the blood
and its distribution, by means of the arteries, to the very extremities

[18] *Ibid.,* chap. iii.
[14] *Ibid.,* chap. iv.
[15] *Ibid.,* chap. v.

of the body; so that the pulse which we feel in the arteries is nothing more than the impulse of the blood derived from the heart.

This statement for its time was tremendous, not a mere revolution, but a genuine innovation.

Harvey's argument now forged forward. If what he had shown concerning the physiology of the heart was sound, why had it remained difficult, he asked, to recognize the rest of the mechanism devoted to a satisfactory blood-flow. The answer was simplicity itself. It must be that the heart and lungs are crowded into such close contact that it becomes difficult to observe what their topographical relations actually are. The pulmonary artery and the pulmonary veins are obviously short and are too soon lost in the substance of the lungs. This fact was his point of departure; he was now ready to discuss the pulmonary circuit. He described the difficulty of the ancients in searching for a passage from pulmonary artery to left ventricle. They searched for it consciously and conscientiously, just as his own countrymen searched for the Northwest passage. Finding none, they necessarily invented pores through the septum. But there were no pores, and there were theoretical objections anyway against their existence.

Harvey sought the pathway by other methods. He resorted to comparative anatomy and found in amphibians and reptiles, which had lungs, and in fish, which had one ventricle but no lungs, what he wanted. What he found was that blood flowed from veins to arteries *through the heart;* the heart itself was the sought-for corridor. And so the physiological Northwest passage was discovered, a quite different proof from that of Servetus! For the same purpose he examined embryos, and found the same thing. Blood passed from the veins into the right ventricle, then through the *foramen ovale* and the *ductus arteriosus* directly into the aorta, obviously *not* through the lungs. He next asked: If this passage exists when the lungs are absent, why does it not do so when they are present and also in use?

To show that this might be so, he relied on argument by anology: water, for example, percolated through the earth, it percolated through the skin, and large quantities taken at spas were known to pass through the parenchyma of the liver and kidneys. If passage through these was possible, why might not blood percolate through the more spongy tissues of the lungs? There was another point which made this passage even more credible, for the liver, being at rest, exercised no propelling force on the blood, whereas the lungs, through their constant motion, were capable of doing so. This was what Columbus thought; this was what Harvey also thought. But for those "who admit nothing unless upon authority," he introduced a passage from Galen which states that the blood *may* so pass and "that this is effected by the ceaseless pulsation of the heart and the motions of the lungs in breathing." [16] Harvey summarizes this and several other passages by saying:

From Galen, however, that great man, that father of physicians, it clearly appears that the blood passes through the lungs from the pulmonary artery into the minute branches of the pulmonary veins, urged to this both by the pulses of the heart and by the motions of the lungs and thorax; . . .[17]

The proof of the pulmonary circuit rests, then, on evidence gathered from comparative anatomy, from dissection of the fetus, and on the inference that what is true of the fetus is also true of the adult, except that the way of the blood after birth is not direct from ventricle to ventricle, but indirect through the lungs. The left ventricle suffices "for the distribution of the blood over the body . . . the right is made for the sake of the lungs, and for the transmission of the blood through them, not for their nutrition." Both ventricles have the same, not different, functions. And so perished another ancient concept. Having settled the problem of the pulmonary passage, Harvey was ready to write his celebrated Eighth Chapter.

The argument had proceeded so far by simple demonstration or on the authority of Galen or of Columbus. But "when," said he, "I surveyed my mass of evidence, whether derived from

[16] Harvey, "An Anatomical Disquisition, etc.," p. 42   [17] *Ibid.*, p. 44.

vivisections, and my various reflections on them"; and when, furthermore, he analyzed the heart, its valves, and its vascular attachments; and when, as he says:

I frequently and seriously bethought me, and long revolved in my mind, what might be the quantity of blood which was transmitted, in how short a time its passage might be effected and the like; . . . I began to think whether there might not be A MOTION, AS IT WERE, IN A CIRCLE.

This was the point, out at last, to which he had been leading. The heart was truly a tremendous organ, "the beginning of life; the sun of the microcosm, even as the sun in his turn might well be designated the heart of the world."

Harvey had now to co-ordinate his several cardinal ideas—the assumption about the circular motion, the province of the heart, the difference between arteries and veins in structure and function—and to proceed to the proof. The argument now became simpler and swifter. He had just spoken of "the quantity of blood which was transmitted"; quantity was the chief consideration in his proof or the one at least which apparently attained the greatest prominence in his mind. The use of quantity was new in physiology. One cannot avoid the insistent question: Did he learn the method in Padua or was it the result of his own devices? Without doubt the method was in the air, for Borelli, who developed it, one might say almost too well, was already twenty years old when Harvey published his treatise. Harvey argued as follows: If the left ventricle post-mortem contains two ounces when dilated, and of course much less when contracted, and expels from a fourth to an eighth of this, that is to say, something between a drachm and a half ounce, then the total expelled in a half hour would range from ten and a half to forty-one and a half pounds. Were it the case of a sheep or dog, a scruple would be expelled, which would amount to three and a half pounds—more in both cases than the whole body contains. These, as later calculations have shown, are relatively small quantities but obviously they are quantities which could not have been ingested nor could they have been drawn from the veins; there can be no escape, therefore, on this ground alone from the conclusion that the blood circulates. Although he believed there was usually great constancy in the volume output, this changed according to age, temperament, sleep, rest, food, exercise, and affections of the mind.

It had now been adequately demonstrated that blood passed from veins to arteries by way of heart and lungs. It was necessary next to show that the circuit was completed *at the periphery* by the reverse passage, from arteries to veins. From the fact that the body could be drained of blood by dividing an artery, a fact well known to Galen and even to Erasistratus, the conclusion had been drawn that anastomoses exist.

That the blood leaves the heart by the arteries and returns to it by the veins and "that the blood passes from the arteries into the veins, and not from the veins into the arteries, and that there is either an anastomosis of the two orders of vessels, or pores in the flesh and solid parts generally that are permeable to blood," [18] Harvey proved by the famous experiment with tight and middle-tight ligatures about the arms. First, with *tight* ones, flow into the arms through the arteries was blocked; these became distended above, while below pulsation ceased. Flow in the veins was also blocked. There was consequently no flow in and no flow out of the extremity. Second, with a *moderately tight one,* matters were different: the arteries continued to pulsate, but the veins now were distended below. When this ligature was undone, the individual experienced a somewhat cold feeling making its way upward. Third, if a *tight ligature was loosened* and the artery palpated, "the blood will be felt to glide through" and the individual experienced a sensation of warmth. Obviously, then, blood flowed into the arm through the arteries, and out through the veins. Fourth, that blood flowed from the arteries into the veins was proved by studying the case of the moderately tight ligature when pulsation of the arteries persisted—that is to say, when blood still entered—but was prevented from flowing out of the arm so that the veins swelled below the ligature. All this, noted Harvey,

[18] Harvey, "An Anatomical Disquisition, etc.," p. 58.

resulted from "the forcing power of the heart" and not at all from heat, pain, or *vis vacui*. There was surely then a passage from arteries to veins.

Harvey next employed the striking proof derived from his study of the venous valves, the one he communicated to Boyle. "Their office," said he, "is by no means explained when we are told that it is to hinder the blood, by its weight, from all flowing into inferior parts; for the edges of the valves in the jugular veins hang downward, and are so contrived that they prevent the blood from rising upwards." The valves all look "invariably towards the seat of the heart." As a matter of fact, he believed that "the valves are solely made and instituted lest the blood should pass from the greater into the lesser veins." He arrived at this belief from his effort to pass probes, which were uniformly blocked when directed from center to periphery. This observation led him on to the four beautiful experiments on the superficial veins of the arm. Lay on a moderately tight ligature. Press one index finger upon a vein and with the other index finger stroke the vein upward to the next valve. You will see first that the interval becomes empty, and second that it cannot be filled from above, even by stroking downward; the valve, you will learn, is tight. Then came the third phase: if you lift the compressing finger, blood flows into the empty vein, not from above, but, you may be quite sure, from below. Finally, if you repeat the first phase—that is to say, compressing and stroking upward—one thousand times in succession and estimate the quantity of blood so allowed to pass upward, "you will find that so much blood has passed through a certain portion of the vessel; and I do now believe that you will find yourself convinced of the circulation of the blood, and of its rapid motion." [19]

Harvey must now be permitted to summarize his case:

Since all things, both argument and ocular demonstration, show that the blood passes through the lungs and heart by the action of the (auricles and) ventricles, and is sent for distribution to all parts of

[19] Harvey, "An Anatomical Disquisition, etc.," p. 67.

the body, where it makes its way into the veins and pores of the flesh, and then flows by the veins from the circumference on every side to the centre, from the lesser to the greater veins, and is by them finally discharged into the vena cava and right auricle of the heart, and this in such a quantity or in such a flux and reflux thither by the arteries, hither by the veins, as cannot possibly be supplied by the ingesta, and is much greater than can be required for mere purposes of nutrition; it is absolutely necessary to conclude that the blood in the animal body is impelled in a circle, and is in a state of ceaseless motion; that this is the act or function which the heart performs by means of its pulse; and that it is the sole and only end of the motion and contraction of the heart.[20]

The formal demonstration was now complete. Harvey had brought to light the function of the heart and its dominant place in the circulation of the blood. But from his own point of view, his task was not yet finished. Traditional physiology ascribed other activities to the heart to which he was obliged also to turn his attention. In tracing their origin and in appraising the meaning of them, it is a great pleasure to me to acknowledge the guiding hand of my own teacher in physiology, Professor John G. Curtis, whose book,[21] prepared after his death with rare devotion and judgment by Professor Lee, is, I may say (I hope without exaggeration), the most scholarly and penetrating study of Harvey's thought which has so far been undertaken.

These other functions Harvey turned then to consider. The primacy of the heart as against the blood, of the blood as against the heart, this old Aristotle-Galen controversy Harvey could not dismiss, even from a treatise so mechanistically conceived as his *De motu cordis*. He felt obliged to consider:

Wherefore does it [that is, the heart] first acquire consistency, and appear to possess life, motion, sense, before any other part of the body is perfected, as Aristotle says in his third book, De partibus Animalium? And so also of the blood: Wherefore does it precede all the rest? And in what way does it possess the vital and animal principle? And show

[20] *Ibid.*, p. 68.
[21] *Harvey's Views on the Use of the*   *Circulation of the Blood*, New York, 1915.

a tendency to motion, and to be impelled hither and thither, the end for which the heart appears to be made? [22]

This was one of the questions about which his views fluctuated, as many references that might be cited show, both in *De motu cordis* and in *De generatione*. But against Galen he takes his place definitely beside Aristotle:

Nor are we the less to agree with Aristotle in regard to the sovereignty of the heart; nor are we to inquire whether it receives sense and motion from the brain? whether blood from the liver? whether it be the origin of the veins and of the blood? and more of the same description. They who affirm these propositions against Aristotle, overlook, or do not rightly understand the principal argument, to the effect that the heart is the first part which exists, and that it contains within itself blood, life, sensation, motion, before either the brain or the liver were in being, or had appeared distinctly, or, at all events, before they could perform any function. The heart, ready furnished with its proper organs of motion, like a kind of internal creature, is of a date anterior to the body: first formed, nature willed that it should afterwards fashion, nourish, preserve, complete the entire animal, as its work and dwelling place: the heart, like the prince in a kingdom, in whose hands lie the chief and highest authority, rules over all; it is the original and foundation from which all power is derived, on which all power depends in the animal body. [23]

There can be no doubt that Harvey was a confirmed Aristotelian. Did he not say in his old age ". . . the authority of Aristotle has always such weight with me that I never think of differing from him inconsiderately." He will appear in the end, however, in *De generatione*, to have indicated his preference for the blood as the prime mover, deducing his proof from the hibernation of certain animals, and of others with blood but without a pulse. [24] The attribution of primacy to the blood is not, however, to be viewed as a capitulation to Galen. Mechanically the heart had been immovably intrenched.

Although formulated later than his treatise of 1628, Harvey's

---

[22] "An Anatomical Disquisition, etc.," p. 74.

[23] *Ibid.*, p. 83.

[24] *Ibid.*, p. 76, ll. 11-29, and p. 374, ll. 28-35.

view of the cause of the heartbeat is interesting, and in a sense completes his account of the mechanism of the heart's motion. He says, ". . . I view the native or innate heat as the common instrument of every function, the prime cause of the pulse among the rest. This, however, I do not mean to state absolutely, but only propose it by way of thesis." [25] By swelling rhythmically at the caval entrance, the auricles, and then the rest of the motion of the heartbeat, are set into action. It is as Curtis says: "The Harveian heart-beat is caused and initiated by an Aristotelian swelling up of the hot blood." [26] Harvey forgot a fact that he himself had adduced, namely, that fragments of muscle and the empty heart, even when taken outside the body, may both contract rhythmically.[27]

In discussing the pulmonary circuit of the blood, it will be remembered that Harvey put the function of the respiration aside, as a subject apart from his present problem. To learn his later views, his other writings must be consulted. The idea of the cooling and tempering effect of the inspired air on the innate heat when taken into the blood and the heart he inherited from Hippocrates, from Aristotle, and from Galen. Aristotle has been at pains to indicate how this was accomplished. He believed that the branches of the trachea were disposed so that they lay parallel in the lungs with the pulmonary vessels and that they held this position because ". . . no common (communicating) channel exists, for it is by contact that they receive the breath and transmit it to the heart." [28] This doctrine of cooling Harvey accepted at first. There was a second ancient doctrine, Galenic rather than Aristotelian, which stated that the air or that part of it which entered the lungs was worked up, or concocted, there first, next in the heart, and in the arteries with that air, in addition, which permeates the skin, and finally with a fresh supply of air in the *rete mirabile* at the base of the brain. This substance became vital spirits in the lungs and heart and animal or psychic spirits in the brain. Natural spirits brought from the right heart by the pul-

[25] *Ibid.*, p. 138.
[26] Curtis, *op. cit.*, p. 90.
[27] Harvey, *op. cit.*, p. 28.

[28] Curtis, *op. cit.*, p. 15; Aristotle, *History of Animals*, 496a, 27-32.

monary artery to the lungs received there their first refinement. It was precisely in discovering that the pulmonary circuit served this function of bringing blood to the lungs to be concocted, wherein Columbus's achievement consisted.

At first Harvey accepted both these doctrines: the doctrine of cooling and the doctrine of concoction, which we now call oxidation. The doctrine of concoction he came later to deny, although it had had adherents for two thousand years and was again adopted soon after his death by Lower. His denial should, however, be credited to Harvey as a virtue, for, relying as he did on the senses, he could adduce no evidence in favor of this mechanism. He could find air neither in the pulmonary artery nor in the left ventricle, even after blowing up the lungs of a dog with a bellows. The difference in color between arterial and venous bloods, which should have aided him, he knew. It would be said now to be as good a guide to the function of oxidation as were the venous valves to the existence of the circulation. He knew the difference—indeed, it had long been known—but he chose to ignore it as being slight and of no account. He came to this conclusion reluctantly because both bloods retained the same volume and assumed an identical color soon after being shed. Of the meaning and origin of spirits he came finally to have doubt. "Spirits," Harvey concluded, are "not from the air." [29] In his old age he came to deny even the cooling effects of the air:

If anyone will carefully attend to these circumstances, and consider a little more closely the nature of air, he will, I think, allow that air is given neither for the "cooling" nor the nutrition of animals; for it is an established fact, that if the foetus has once respired, it may be more quickly suffocated than if it had been entirely excluded from the air. . . . As the arguments on either side are very equally balanced, it is a question of the greatest difficulty. [30]

And so the matter ended, without decision. He tried out the theories of the ancients and found them wanting. Unlike the one into which the capillaries later fitted, he recognized no new assumption concerning the respiration that he could make either

[29] Curtis, *op. cit.*, p. 34.   [30] Harvey, *op. cit.*, p. 530.

in regulating the temperature or in providing a mechanism for oxidation.

Harvey's work was done. He had been inducted into the anatomical tradition at Cambridge; he became absorbed in anatomical problems at Padua; he practiced anatomical investigation in London. Throughout his life he was devoted to a problem, interest in which began in Greece, and was transferred successively to Alexandria, to Pergamum, to Paris, and to Padua, in the end to come upon its final study and solution in England. It was the outstanding physiological problem of the classical world. This he inherited as all scientists inherit their problems except that in this case knowledge had already attained advanced development. He absorbed and mastered its entire literature, and he unraveled completely its intricate nature. Its complexity was not less great than the problem studied by Kepler; Harvey, too, was required to deal with many factors incredibly difficult to understand. To each he gave new functions, ordered them all in a simplified organism, and achieved a synthesis not only unified but aesthetically satisfying.

What Harvey achieved is acknowledged by universal assent to be the foundation for further development. Whether that development necessarily sprang from what he actually accomplished is more doubtful. From the oft-repeated statement that this discovery began a new era in physiology, it seems necessary to dissent. Nutrition and respiration became the outstanding subjects of investigation in the new era. The birth of psychology has been delayed until our own day. The study of the respiration remained deadlocked even though Lower, eight years after Harvey's death, found the clue here to the difference in the color of the two bloods. A complete solution necessarily awaited the satisfactory development and appreciation of chemistry. This way Mayow lighted, though the leaders of the Royal Society failed to see it. Then the vogue of Stahl completely obscured it. Van Helmont and Black, Priestley and Lavoisier, one hundred and fifty years after the publication of *De motu cordis* finally discovered it and followed along Mayow's way. Lavoisier saw the way chemically at once, but it was even later that oxidation was transferred from the lungs to the tissues. Then it was that the long inquiry terminated, so checkered in its course from Aristotle and Hippocrates to Galen, from Galen to Harvey, from Harvey to Lower. This is not the history characteristic of a discovery that initiates a new era. It is more just to regard Harvey's great achievement as the close, not the beginning of a period. He stands, not in time but in thought, midway between the ancient and the modern worlds.

No one who is in a moderate degree historically minded and interested in the evolution of the human intellect can escape reflecting on, and attempting to appraise Harvey's place in the scientific movement of the Renaissance. I find myself adhering quite naturally to a statement Mr. H. O. Taylor recently made:

We bear in mind that physical science, and each branch of it, is a unity and a whole, made of its present and its past; so that the history of any science is verily that science itself in its entirety and continuous course from its beginning to what it is now and hereafter shall come to be.[31]

No clearer example than Harvey can be furnished in evidence of this conception; he has himself amply demonstrated its truth in the course of his own writings. He summed up in its entirety the history of his science. Of his relation to his contemporaries of the 17th Century it is more difficult to speak. The record is lamentably vague. What there is of it gives the impression of a far greater continuity with the past than of intimate sympathy with his own world. His ever-present intellectual companions were Aristotle and Galen. His correspondence, so much of it as has been preserved, is exasperatingly slight. In his writings there is no mention of a single contemporary English author, certainly a remarkable fact at the end of the age of Elizabeth. The single poetical quotation in *De motu cordis* is taken from Terence. That with men like Winston, professor of physic at Gresham College, he had little basis for companionship is no surprise. But Gilbert was still alive when he returned from Padua; and the group of

[31] "A Layman's View of History," *American Historical Review*, 1928, XXXIII, 252.

inquiring intellects—Hooke, Wren, Boyle, Petty—which formed the Royal Society three years after his death, had been actively gathering during the last seventeen years of his life at meetings centered around Gresham College, at the time the most interesting experiment in scientific education. With none of these men does he seem to have established relations of friendship, but rather with Thomas Hobbes who attacked them as anti-Aristotelians. Robert Boyle, that extraordinarily curious and inquiring mind, met him only once, and that shortly before Harvey's death, when Boyle was already thirty years old. There was no companionship that is traceable now which can be said to have been stimulating or to have influenced significantly the course of his thought. He must have been a person singularly devoted to his special interests, little concerned with the problems of the scientific world that surrounded him. Of chemists and of chemistry, Aubrey tells us that he held a poor opinion. And of Galilei, who was making Padua alive with curiosity in subjects of really great general concern, and whose lecture-room adjoined that of Fabricius so that Harvey could scarcely have escaped seeing him, we catch no echo in his writing. There is no reason to believe that what Galilei had to say had much interest for him, although many an Englishman on his grand tour must have sought him out as had John Milton. He was unsympathetic to Galilei, as later to Aselli: ". . . no kind of science can possibly flow," said Harvey, "save from some pre-existing knowledge of more obvious things; and this is one main reason why our science in regard to the nature of celestial bodies, is so uncertain and conjectural." [32] There is, indeed, an animadversion against the new astronomy in that same treatise in which he says: ". . . and there are persons who will not be content to take up with a new system, unless it explains everything, as in astronomy." [33] When, in point of fact, Harvey turned away from anatomy to find a metaphor for the circle in which the blood travels, he turned not to the new science but back to Aristotle, and remarked: "Which motion we may be allowed to call circular,

[32] Harvey, *A Second Disquisition to Riolanus; in Which Many Objections to* *the Circulation of the Blood Are Refuted*, p. 132.

[33] *Op. cit.*, p. 123.

in the same way as Aristotle says that the air and the rain emulate the circular motion of the superior bodies; . . ." [34] For mathematics, however, he developed a deep interest, especially in his declining years. He mastered Oughtred's *Clavis mathematicae* and was working problems from it not long before he died.

There are those who profess not to rate high this achievement of Harvey. It lacks experimental elaborateness and the complicated and dazzling procedures of the modern laboratory. But if he is the great scientist who possesses a capacious mind, who sees his problem and who sees it whole, who bends his energy to its solution, and who in his demonstration exhibits that fine aesthetic quality which restrains exuberance and limits his proof to what is relevant, then I have no hesitation in linking the name of Harvey with that enviable company of which Kepler and Newton, Lamarck and Darwin, are the shining examples.

I have come to the end of my analysis. It has been the record of a great history in which the intellectual giants of the race have taken their part. Neither Aristotle nor Galen needs my praise. But although not the heroes of my story, I am reluctant to part company with them without dwelling on the distinction of their contributions to the ultimate solution of this problem. The more theirs appear to be internally coherent, the greater is the credit due to Harvey, who saw that what he received from them was a thing of fragments. He inherited a heart which did not work, anastomoses which did not exist, pores in the ventricular septum which would not die, vessels which knew no consistency of motion. Into the heart he breathed energy; into the vascular system, order. One, certainly, of the most complex mechanisms in nature attained in his capacious intellect completely harmonious arrangement. To have brought about this innovation represents one of the great somersaults in the history of the human understanding.

[34] Harvey, "An Anatomical Disquisition, etc.," p. 46.

On Simon Flexner: 1863-1946

Y EARS ago I had the singular opportunity of introducing one of my friends and associates to Simon Flexner. That friend was A. Samoiloff, Professor of Physiology at the University of Samara, at that time called Kazan. We had, I thought, a good, though a somewhat formal, talk. It must have been about professional matters. After an appropriate time we left and, the weather being fine, sauntered out into the yard of the Institute. In good, continental fashion, Samoiloff stopped, faced me, took me by the arm, and said "Aber, Herr Kollege, dass ist ein Minister." Anyone familiar with officialdom will know what Samoiloff meant.

During the war, it must have been about 1914, Keith (Sir Arthur Keith) Curator of the Royal College of Surgeons, came to New York to see to it that all was right with the United States. It had been my privilege and pleasure to be allowed to examine in Keith's museum hearts which exhibited congenital malformations. I took him to call on Dr. Flexner. This was a warmer talk. That may have been because Keith also was an official. Being early in the history of institutes especially designed to carry on research, how to arrange for their continuity and undiminished efficiency occupied everybody's mind interested in such matters. Clearly it was in Dr. Flexner's—perhaps at the top of it. And certainly it interested Keith, for in England thinking in these directions was scarcely even in its infancy. The north windows of Dr. Flexner's study looked out upon the old Power House of The Rockefeller Institute which already, after only ten years, was aging. Additional buildings were then in the blue-print stage. During the conversation Dr. Flexner beckoned Keith to his window and explained that ruthlessness was the core of the business of providing continuity. It was not necessary to be sentimental about that Power House. When it ceased to serve its function it would be scrapped and replaced by a better. This was a metaphor. After a while Keith and I left. This had been no "interview" but a meeting. I was at that time young at the Institute and very junior. As we neared the door Dr. Flexner put his arm about my shoulder and said, "I didn't mean you."

In 1920, at the end of the war, when Dr. Meltzer had retired and chemotherapy was young, Dr. Flexner made a voyage to Europe to study the effects of the war on the medical sciences, and took me with him so that I might join in writing a report of what men interested in pharmacology seemed to be thinking—we wanted guides for our own development. One morning aboard ship he suddenly appeared outside the window of my cabin on the promenade deck, while I was shaving, stuck his head in and uttered a single syllable—"Boo." Then followed a discussion on the advantage of safety razors. I was wielding a straight one. I still do.

Simon Flexner made it easy for people to misunderstand him. He could be official, and often was. He could appear ruthless—a Director needed to be—but in his heart that is not what he was. He could be playful, but I fear few people saw him as I had the good fortune to do, as an easy-going agreeable companion. His interests were broadly humane. He was interested in *the* people—but not in miscellaneous people. What everyone to whom he owed responsibility knew was that he was a man of infinite considerateness, of affectionate disposition, and solicitous for the welfare of persons dependent on him. Because he had this range and his gift, or need, for anonymity, it should not be unexpected that men differ sharply about what nature of man he actually was. It is too soon and the material at anyone's disposal, certainly mine, is too slim to offer anything resembling a full and correct picture of him. These are very personal recollections of the man. I think he was a great man.

It was my opportunity on a few occasions to know something of what agitated his mind concerning the future of The Rockefeller Institute and its place in the world. He did not think The Rockefeller Institute could be isolated. Whatever his thought concerning that place may have been, he would have been the first to say, he had no intention, nor was he interested in finding, a background either in systematic theory, in historical evolution or in philosophical perspective for what he wished to accomplish. He was a man who read biographies, not often history and less often still works of general or philosophical inquiry. For him science meant opportunity. And the opportunities that were to be seized were the opportunities of today. His was a concrete mind, dealing with concrete phenomena, projecting concrete futures not intended, in his judgment, to serve any but a limited scope.

In the end, and this is the burden of my testimony, this way of his of looking, apparently so circumscribed, aided in changing the complexion of the intellectual scientific life of three continents. If he began by being ambitious merely for himself, though with no great sense of achieving his personal fame, what he accomplished was enlargement of the scientific horizon, notably in the United States. If President Gilman was the chief instrument in that adventure before 1900, I think it is not unfair to claim for Simon Flexner the next great forward step afterward. He stood on a watershed on one side of which was the intellectual achievement which centered in the creation and early years of the Johns Hopkins University and on the other what became of that promise after the founding of the Institute. There can be no doubt that the ideas which germinated in Baltimore fell like the mantle of Elijah, a forced simile this, upon the shoulders of the Institute in New York.

The significant characteristic of the Institute is the very concreteness which was so congenial to Dr. Flexner. Here was uncovered a way of arranging an environment in which ideas could be made to grow. Science in the United States could not escape pointing the way of that growth. If its beginnings were meager and hard and had their roots in Europe, even if the very men who carried on that work were European, the exuberant wealth of the country disposed it to this inevitable evolution when it came, intellectually, of age.

I remember, being an alumnus of Columbia College and Columbia University, a report, current at the time, that President

Butler could not understand why, when The Rockefeller Institute was founded, a separate institution needed to be created. Why could it not become part of his university? Why could he not, thought I at the time, have thought of this himself and have made the University great and forestalled the development of such institutions as The Rockefeller Institute, to say nothing of the great expansion of industrial research for which subsequently homes were found in the research laboratories of the great corporations? These questions raise interesting problems. And they have great importance too, for the growth of the country. But these are better treated somewhere else.

I mentioned the fact just now that Europeans constituted the nucleus of men of science, if not in the country, certainly in The Rockefeller Institute. The staff in the first few years consisted of Samuel Meltzer, a Russian, P. A. Levene, a Russian, Jacques Loeb, an Alsatian German, Alexis Carrel, a Frenchman. Of native Americans between 1904 and 1909 Dr. Flexner and Dr. Eugene Opie were the only ones. There were six [1] other men on the staff, but none of them became permanent members.

It must have been the composition of this dramatis personae and his deep desire to think out ways of continuing the early achievement and securing its leadership that suggested to Dr. Flexner a very ingenious plan. There were undoubtedly relatively few persons in the country available for appointment to the Institute. He was always on the watch for them. He tried them out in junior positions. The device he was looking for must be of a nature to encourage the development of the persons the Institute needed. He found that device. I think that in this he was a step in advance of President Gilman. Gilman sought and found men, but aside from the usual facilities a university offered he made no effort to create them.

Dr. Flexner's was a method, as one looks back, eminently characteristic of him. He did not like to show his hand. He chanced—indeed it was no chance but one of the inevitabilities—

[1] J. E. Sweet, E. H. Eising, W. A. Beatty, H. S. Houghton, J. W. Jobling and J. Auer. Dr. Opie withdrew in 1909.

to be a Member of the Board of The Rockefeller Foundation. He was in fact a Charter Member and one of its Incorporators in 1913. Mr. Raymond Fosdick told us in his Memorial Address that he was the accepted dean of that Board. It was, Mr. Fosdick still thinks, a board of giants. Dr. Flexner was its chief scientific adviser. In 1919 the Foundation began to put at the disposal of the National Research Council sums of money to make possible the education of Fellows. Several millions of dollars have been appropriated for this purpose.

"The first series of these fellowships was inaugurated in 1919 for physics and chemistry, and was later extended to include mathematics and astronomy." [2]

The plan so initiated and developed was designed to accomplish the ends Dr. Flexner had in view. The Fellows were men who already had been granted the degree of Doctor of Philosophy or Doctor of Medicine. They were not young or wholly untried persons. They were eligible to 35, in some cases to 40 years. They were men who had already given evidence of their powers and intentions. These were the men to whom Fellowships were offered. The conditions were extremely liberal—in the size of stipends, the length of holidays, the supply of equipment. The Fellows were encouraged to study under masters best suited to their purposes. They were in a large sense free men. An appointment for three years could be renewed another three; a person could obviously be carried along until it was all but certain that he would succeed. Fellows could study at home or abroad. And they did—322 (25%) went abroad. There are chemists and physicists—biochemists and bio-physicists, biologists, geneticists and physiologists. Their number must rapidly have increased, their abilities have been great, their locations by appointment throughout the country, many and varied. It would be not uninteresting to learn the degree of success and distinction to which individuals attained. It would no doubt turn out to be a notable company.

This was the group of men Dr. Flexner's plan created. It was

[2] *National Research Fellowships 1919-1944.* Administered by the National Research Council, Washington, D. C., June 30, 1944.

a patriotic scheme serviceable not only in the great world outside but also in the smaller world of the Institute. But whether these men became available to The Rockefeller Institute made little difference. In point of fact fifty Fellows earned the opportunity to work there. One of them became a Member and three, Associate Members of the Institute. The country could not fail to benefit from the abundance of men of so much superior competence. The Institute and the country—both benefited from this large, imaginative patriotism.

There have been those, and they are many, who have never thought of Dr. Flexner in any other sense than as Director of The Rockefeller Institute. With this he has been identified to such a degree that his significance in the larger world has often been missed. When the whole story is told it will turn out, I believe, that this is too small a view to take of his extraordinary contribution to science in general. How the scheme of the National Research Fellowships actually worked these few statistics demonstrate:

Until 1944-45 1,289 Fellows had been appointed.

In the Physical Sciences	.	.	.	530
" " Geography and Geology	.	.	13
" " Medical Sciences	.	.	319
" " Biological Sciences	.	.	427
			1289 *

* Before deduction of one name registered in two groups.

His contact in England with men who were in charge of furthering the interests of medical research began early. Abraham Flexner tells the story of having met Mr. Lloyd George at luncheon at Sir Michael Sadler's in Oxford in 1927-28. Lloyd George recalled an early meeting with Dr. Flexner: "I saw your brother (Simon) 10 or 12 years before that, when I was Chancellor of the Exchequer. . . . I can tell you exactly what we talked about, namely, certain features of the Insurance Bill which I was piloting through the House of Commons.[3] That must have

[3] *I Remember,* The Autobiography of Abraham Flexner, New York, 1940.

been in 1908 or 1909. Their topic must have been the Medical Research Council and its very important furthering of medical research in Great Britain.

Those were exciting days not only in England but everywhere else where the need to further the interests of medicine was understood. There in England were the beginnings of devoting money taken from taxation for the advancement of learning in the interest of the people. About that need Lloyd George was clear. The precise organization changed subsequently, but government as the source of such support seems to have been laid securely at that time. With that sophistication which is characteristic of British administration, reflecting on how this money was to be spent occupied a great deal of time. Ways needed to be found in which this could be done without prejudice to academic initiative, freedom and organization. A distinguished scientist was the first administrator of this fund. Sir Walter Fletcher had before this become a significant investigator and was known throughout the world of physiology because of his joint researches with Professor, later Sir, F. Gowland Hopkins. Lloyd George discussed, as I have said, features of this problem with Dr. Flexner. It chanced to be my good fortune, much later, in 1920, to be present at discussions between Dr. Flexner and Sir Walter. I confess to my own lack of foresight. I was unaware that I was a part, even if only an onlooker, of great things in the making. I took no notes. I do not recollect the precise topics under discussion at one, to me nevertheless, memorable dinner. That I cannot recite upon this may be a great loss. But the time and the fact that I was included suggest that the discussion must have touched upon the development of university hospitals and hospitals at which medical investigation was to be carried on, much as was already being done at The Rockefeller Institute.

For this was about the time when the great clinical research units were established in London, at the London Hospital, at University College, at St. Bartholomew's and at Guy's Hospitals. The conception of that kind of research in hospitals was one which had its slow growth first in the United States. Had there been no other way it could not fail to have been imported into Great

Britain and communicated to the authorities in England when two physicians, Francis R. Fraser and Arthur Ellis, one a Scot and the other a Canadian, were chosen to be heads of the units.[4] These two men both received their scientific clinical training in The Hospital of the Rockefeller Institute. It was very natural that they should turn out to be links in the transatlantic chain that bound our two countries in this kind of comradeship. These were years in point of fact in which, through frequent interchange, British to the United States and Americans to Britain, communication took place thick and fast. Service with the British of many distinguished American physicians in World War I laid the foundations of many intimacies. This occurred especially in the Base Hospitals. It was in fact my own responsibility to nominate specialists in cardiac diseases for Thomas Lewis. He trained them in the memorable institution at Colchester. That experience opened the way for Lewis's subsequent fame in the United States.

There is a way of regarding Simon Flexner as central to this development. Being Director he did in the first place aid powerfully in creating an environment in which this kind of research was recognized as being needed. It began first in the independent laboratories of the Institute. They followed the continental model. But then, soon after founding the laboratories, the plan to further scientific research was built (1910) into the new hospital as the indispensable method for studying diseases. Developing side by side the ancillary sciences and the study of diseases aided and fructified each other. In a world of shifting ideas the precise designations of disciplines, pure and impure science, will also shift. What was essential was recognition of the fact that to gain knowledge of diseases it was valuable to house patients who suffered from them in such a fashion as to make possible investigations as careful as was already possible in simpler situations in the natural sciences. The new hospital was, it need scarcely be said, an ex-

[4] Fraser's coming to The Rockefeller Institute was a chance. Dr. Flexner was visiting his father, Sir Thomas Fraser, Professor of Clinical Medicine in Edinburgh. He mentioned Fraser's plan of going to Germany for his further training. Dr. Flexner then described the new opportunity in New York. Young Fraser journeyed West, instead of East, with results of great import.

pansion quite unique. The fact that in Germany men like Wunderlich and Traube furnished laboratories in a somewhat peripheral way does not make less the significance or revolutionary character of the new development here.

Rufus Cole, the first Director of The Hospital of the Rockefeller Institute, wrote: "Laboratories of a primitive character began to be established. in the clinics, in Munich in 1886, in Leipzig in 1892, and in the United States, in the Johns Hopkins Hospital, opened in 1889. The chief object of these laboratories, however, was the improvement of diagnosis." ". . . thoughtful physicians came to realize that in order really to understand disease and to perfect rational measures of treatment, more refined methods of investigation were required." [5] The word "rational" should not be passed over lightly. When Abraham Flexner's recollection of Mr. Lloyd George's conversations with Dr. Flexner is recalled and when it is remembered that, at about the same time the university hospitals, first at the Johns Hopkins University, began to be established in the United States; and when, furthermore, the significant role which Mr. Flexner played through his reports to the Carnegie Corporation (1910 and 1912) on medical education both in the United States and in Europe is added, the chances are good that a shrewd guess would indicate the nature of Dr. Flexner's role in the furtherance of the entire enterprise.

Later Dr. Flexner was appointed Eastman Visiting Professor at Oxford in the academic year 1937-38. Eastman Professors are Americans. They owe their selection not to their ability to carry on formal instruction, but to their ability to make possible frequent informal and intimate discussions of academic problems in their own professions. This was the time when plans for utilizing the large and significant gifts from Lord Nuffield to strengthen the medical establishments in Oxford were being made. Those who were responsible for developing them naturally thought of Dr. Flexner as that representative of the recent American advances who could be of greatest usefulness as counsellor. Toward the

[5] *Forschungsinstitute; ihre Geschichte, Organisation und Ziele,* L. Brauer, A. M. Bartholdy and A. Meyer, Hamburg, 1930, p. 491.

middle of his residence he delivered two lectures, on January 20 and 27, 1938, entitled "The Evolution and Organization of the University Clinic." The lecture itself is rich and allusive dealing as it does with many phases of the problems immediately at issue. The nature of university clinics, he says, "involves three things:

1. The provision of laboratories in the clinic where there can be conducted scientific research equal in fundamental importance to that carried out by the general laboratories along with the training of students in scientific medicine and its methods.

2. Clinical professors who are qualified in at least one subject of medical research to be both leaders of their research associates and technical workers in one of the several laboratories attached to the clinic.

3. The power of the professor to command his time for the patients from whom the research problems are derived, for the laboratory in which those problems are investigated, and for the teaching of students in the science of their profession.

The key to the achievement of these conditions lies in the laboratories. I venture, therefore, at the outset to place before you in brief and incomplete fashion the history of the development of the laboratory where investigator and student meet and labour together, a development which within the last one hundred years has done more than anything else to give to medicine its scientific character." [6]

An episode which illustrates Dr. Flexner's influence in the development of the sciences is to be found, of all places, in Germany. After having accepted the Directorship of The Rockefeller Institute in 1902, he decided, in 1903, to go abroad. He spent the year with Professor v. Recklinghausen and with Professor Emil Fischer. The period in Fischer's laboratory was peculiarly significant. His reason for being there was his belief that chemistry, especially organic chemistry, was to have signal importance for medical research. He wanted to see, at first hand, how this was being conducted in one of the most distinguished laboratories in the world. In the course of his sojourn in Berlin he came to know Fischer and conversations between them did in fact take place

[6] *The Evolution and Organization of the University Clinic,* Oxford, 1939, pp. 5-6.

concerning Dr. Flexner's plans. He explained to Professor Fischer
what his purposes were at The Rockefeller Institute and this he
must have done so vividly that I remember his once having told
me the gist of one of Fischer's replies. Professor Fischer's comment was in effect that if in the United States a movement like
this was being undertaken, there could be no doubt that with
our energy and our wealth, Germany would be left behind in
the race. Within a reasonable period of time, in 1911, the laboratories of the Kaiser Wilhelm-Gesellschaft took form. What is
known about their origin is amply set forth in Professor Brauer's
Forschungsinstitute; ihre Geschichte, Organisation und Ziele. The
German institutes were eminently successful. Besides those at
Dahlem, at Dortmund and at Heidelberg there were in 1930,
thirty such laboratories devoted to every conceivable scientific
object. What the Germans accomplished alone and with American help is well known.

Perhaps Dr. Flexner's unfolding his plans for The Rockefeller
Institute to Emil Fischer was America's return to the Germans
for Professor Cohnheim's suggestion to President Gilman that
Dr. William H. Welch be made Director of the School of Medicine at the Johns Hopkins University.[7]

As if these were not enough, chance made it possible for Flexner
to make a contribution on the other side of the world. In the 1910s
The Rockefeller Foundation became interested in the possibility
of stimulating the development of science in China. It is not quite
clear in what manner the initiative came to be taken, but Dr.
Flexner was a member of one of the three Commissions which
the Foundation sent to China. The one in 1915 which Dr. Flexner joined had as members, beside himself, Dr. Wallace Buttrick
and Dr. W. H. Welch. Their secretary was young Dr. Gates,
the son of that remarkable Frederick Gates who achieved such
wide and well deserved fame as the elder Mr. Rockefeller's wise
and energetic almoner.

[7] *I Remember.* The Autobiography of
Abraham Flexner, New York, 1940,
pp. 95-96.

The Chinese needed at that time to be brought abreast of the kind of opportunity which had recently become available in the United States and in Europe. Dates, so often despised, are worth noticing. The founding of The Rockefeller Institute took place in 1901, of the Medical Research Committee (Great Britain) in 1911, of the Kaiser Wilhelm-Gesellschaft in 1911, of the Peking Union Medicine College in 1922. Truly the world was "one world" before 1943. China, in the minds of most men, so remote, actually did not lag far behind in the forward march. What was achieved in Peking was the union of already existing medical schools, now to be called the Peking Union Medical College. New buildings were provided for this enterprise. I speak from first-hand knowledge of the representative character of the buildings as symbols of their contemporary purpose. Their architect made the Chinese architectural idiom serve with extraordinary success the purposes of an institution to be devoted to instruction. Syntheses like these have often been attempted with Greek and Roman formulae, but not often has a liveliness been imparted into such structures as resulted in these in Peking. The story was current at the time that Chinese artisans flocked from all over the country—it sounds like a story out of Florence—to work so that they might relate to their grandchildren that they had taken part in creating this milestone along the road of the evolution of Chinese culture. The buildings certainly are things of beauty. They served their purposes too, in anatomy, in physiology, in biology, in immunology, in medicine and surgery as well as did comparable buildings elsewhere. This became one of the best of modern medical schools. To have had to do with this achievement could not fail of being a source of pride. It was not the only one, but it was an outstanding contribution which succeeded in stimulating the imagination of the Chinese on their road to modernity.

There were Chinese upon the faculty from the very beginning. There was also occasionally an undergraduate European or American student. The Chinese are capable of learning and they learned fast. Soon they became professors and were successful as original investigators. The reconstructed China of 1946 will naturally and necessarily take on much greater responsibility than it did a brief 23 years ago.

It could not be otherwise than that the creation of such an institution presented not insuperable but certainly very difficult problems, the most important of which concerned language. The situation was not unlike that which took place in connection with the founding of the Hebrew University in Jerusalem. There too, an ancient language presented difficulties in furthering the interests of a re-born culture. There was of course, and there is, a great difference between the precise problems in Jerusalem and in Peking. For the most part those who were to carry on whatever was planned in Jerusalem were Europeans, familiar with European languages, English, French, German and Italian, long used and made flexible for scientific purposes. The problem in Palestine was to make an old language scarcely alive in any philosophical or scientific sense, serve the purposes of modern science. That language, for scientific purposes, could scarcely be said to have been a going concern at any time. I was present at a dinner to which the late Justice Brandeis invited Dr. Chaim Weizmann, who conceived the idea and very soon the fact of the Hebrew University, and Dr. Flexner for the purpose of discussing its scientific problems. Science in general and the place of science in that university were the central themes. That was in London in 1920. It was an extraordinary occasion. And how strange— "romantic" even more mature persons than school girls would say—the very place names, London, New York, Washington, Jerusalem, Peking, tied together through the interests of these visionaries. I remember with much vividness the play of these remarkable men and the nature of the conversation. It is the more interesting because related to the problems in Peking, already behind him, there ran through Dr. Flexner's thinking a consistency which characterized the clarity of his own view. At that time, I do not know who knew, but certainly Dr. Flexner had no information on the state of development of the Hebrew language. What the situation was, is described in a recent review by Leon Roth, of translations of the great Philosophical Classics into Hebrew by contemporary scholars. The current volumes were published by the Hebrew University Press.[8]

Roth recalls that at the end of the medieval period Hebrew was utilized. It is widely known that it was famous as a vehicle for conveying to European scholars mathematics, medicine, astronomy, alchemy, physics, psychology and folk-lore. There was in fact a Provençal school of translators, he tells us, who saw to it that the language was kept adequate to this purpose. But then its development stopped. Writers who wished to use Hebrew at the end of the 18th Century found that its medieval style and idiom were quite incomprehensible—"bound fast in a terminology fixed by medieval scholasticism"—except to those accustomed to its use. Now, in our day, when contemporary students again have need of Hebrew for philosophical purposes, they find it necessary to bridge a gap of five hundred years. With very good sense the modern translators faced their problem historically. Modern philosophy having begun with Descartes, they began with Descartes. In translating him into Hebrew they remade the language to fit their modern ends. When they refashioned the ancient medium to make it capable of assimilating the beginnings of modern philosophy, these translators moved onward step by step to make it express Leibnitz, Berkeley, Hume and Rousseau. The effort is said to be crowned with success. Whether Hebrew scientists have managed as well in teaching in the Hebrew language, to be articulate in science, I have not learned. But here, at all events, is evidence concerning the state of the language in 1920 when Dr. Flexner was consulted and is justification of the general view which he took.

The problem as he saw it, is better illustrated in connection with the school in Peking. Chinese also is an ancient language expressive of a very old culture. Chinese, as a vernacular, was however a going concern and was already being modernized. If not made for science there was still no problem of reviving a language. The

[8] Philosophical Classics. Vols. 1-22. Jerusalem, Hebrew University Press, reviewed by Leon Roth, in "Books in Review," *Commentary*, June, 1946, p. 298.

problem was to find a means of expressing European ideas in a medium in which such ideas were not in any sense at home. Since its written form was pictographic it was not easy to make it conform to the requirements of Western science. Chinese, if not at once, would very naturally need ultimately to provide a language suitable to the requirements of scientific expression. It could be molded, but not quickly, to scientific purposes. I visited, in 1925 a commission which sat at Tsinan, manufacturing an appropriate vocabulary. I picked up there fascicles of the glossary. Text-books could, of course, be selected and then translated into Chinese. But text-books are not enough. And yet if teaching could be undertaken with these tools, the Chinese would be spared the painful need of adding a European language to their own already difficult education.

Dr. Flexner agreed that this was possible. But he regarded the obstacles so created as insuperable if the Chinese were to become modern scientists. It was, he thought, not merely a question of language and the immediate translation of Western ideas into an unfamiliar, probably still inflexible, medium, but the fact that the world of science would remain shut to the Chinese, nevertheless. Science was European and was written in the languages of Western Europe. All of them contributed to its evolution and all of them grew out of Mediterranean, especially Greco-Roman alphabets. The genius of language has been making a profound impression on the form of Mediterranean thinking. There is without doubt, intimacy in the relation between thought and form—the form, the genius of language. To deprive Chinese students wishing to study science of intimate knowledge of European languages made them run the risk of being excluded from comprehending the very literatures in which those sciences found expression and with which they were to be so vitally concerned. The Chinese were in a worse fix even than the Jews. There was a struggle. In the end Dr. Flexner's insistence carried the day. The Chinese were to have the best the West could bring to them.

We may wonder what would have happened had not the Boxer indemnity been used for educating Chinese in the United States, where they became familiar with English, and had it not been decided to use English and the other European languages to teach science in China. It would certainly have become much more difficult for the Chinese to come abreast of the modern world. It is a fitting speculation how great the influence of language has been, and more especially the English language, during the last 45 years, in the modernization, not to use the harsher word— revolutionization—of the Chinese. The peculiar differences in language, law and custom, between Anglo-America and Western Europe vis-à-vis Russia give point to the nature and difficulty of mutual understanding. The difference in ideas, having arisen in cultures so regionally characteristic, is fostered no doubt by the genius of two languages expressive, geographically and intricately, of two such very different systems. Understanding as well as inter-communication become unavoidably vastly uncertain. Had the Western Greco-Roman tradition gone in Russia through the medium of a Greco-Roman language instead of through an Eastern one, some at least of the tensions of our world would have been released. But this is all commonplace and argument in a circle. Similarity in language carries with it much of similarity in intellectual idiom. What the compulsions are, of forms of expression upon thinking, proposes in itself, if not exactly a practical speculation, an interest of its own.

At all events, in China, Dr. Flexner prevailed. The language of science and especially of medical science has become English. The Chinese by leaps and bounds have become contemporary. They have achieved political sophistication in the Western sense. They were already past masters of it in the Oriental. In medical science, in geology and perhaps in other sciences, they have been brought measurably abreast of conceptions of Western science. So rapid has been their progress they have already made signal contributions to scientific knowledge. The pseudopod of Western culture stretching into China, has made possible forward strides in anthropology to which the cainozoic laboratories at the Peking Union Medical College have contributed. The Chinese have taken part in studies of *homo Chinensis* first under the direction of Davidson Black and then in most distinguished fashion under Professor Weidenreich.

In the minds of his contemporaries Simon Flexner stood forth through his direction of The Rockefeller Institute. Great as that was, he has, as I have been urging, other claims to fame. In the long view his influence on American science and scientific organization, and other activities of his abroad, though they have received less attention, will add to his stature in ways that have been little foreseen. In three continents, what he thought and suggested has accelerated the pace of living. What he did will stand out as fructifying contributions to the enlargement of the scientific spirit. He was a shy man. He believed himself isolated and he walked warily in fostering interests that lay close to his heart. To accomplish an end, he often disappeared behind the scene. He worked through great organizations—The Rockefeller Foundation, the National Research Council, the China Medical Board. His has not been an uncommon device. Significant, forceful and farseeing men have often made it their own.

He was singularly fortunate. The elder Mr. Rockefeller and Mr. Frederick Gates were completely sympathetic to the creation of instruments which made possible the expression of his genius.

Apologia Mea

RECENTLY, our President sent me a copy of President Shuster's contribution to this symposium. I trust I attribute to him not less astuteness than he actually possesses, when I assume he did so to make me aware of the singular charm a spiritual biography can exhibit.

I shall be describing to you in stark language the phases through which my mind has passed in arriving at what it has become. When I began attempting to think of what to impart, I said to myself—what Professor Whitehead once said to me—I do not feel anything going on. Next morning, as I lay contemplating my sense of emptiness, there began suddenly to pour out from my unconscious a stream of recollections which I could not stem. I was thinking back on how it all began and was astonished when I recognized how much, perhaps everything, in the pattern of my mind had been set in my childhood. I was forced to pay tribute to Freud. I had not appreciated how right he is. My unconscious stream presented first of all the image of my maternal grandfather who was President of the Synagogue in Savannah, Georgia. He was kept in office, I recalled, because it was discovered that he was the only man in the State who could blow a shofar. Of course, he read books. It would take a full-dress psychoanalytical history to learn whether the main streams of my subsequent mental life began there. At all events I know nothing now, earlier than this, that has significance, except the fact that he was a soldier of sorts. He became a colonel, an honorary colonel, of the Chatham Artillery, an ancient, perhaps the oldest, military organization in the country, and was buried with military honors. This other trait, inherited from him, accounts for my easily aroused belligerence. Remember, if you please, that Savannah lay in the Rebellion.

Before I go on let me dispose of an important issue. I shall not define what I mean by spiritual until the end when the meaning I assign to reason and rational has become clear and also the meanings of irrational and wilfulness—not quite the same as unreason. You will notice that I do not stop to discuss "beauty" nor the appreciation of beauty, nor Aesthetics as that universe of discourse which concerns itself with these matters. These are secondary Cartesian characteristics. The degree to which I have been sensitive to such impressions is indicated in what I shall say of Professor Woodberry. I ask you to accept the great influence of music and the crafts upon me. Without their influence, existence may have been unbearable.

Our home in New York was middle class and bourgeois. My father immigrated into the country when he was 8 or 9 years old, in about the year 1854. His early life was like that of most immigrants, poor, hard-working, frugal and successful. I have never heard that he passed through anything called a formal education. Later, when I knew him, he was a man of powerful intellect, in economics conventional but intellectually uncompromising. He seceded with Felix Adler from the Temple Emanu-el, that same religious society in New York which now dwells in marble halls, when Dr. Adler founded the Society for Ethical Culture. But he seceded from that too, either because it was too much or because it was not enough. I do not know which. But subsequently he became an unpracticing and I think unbelieving Jew.

It must have been for this reason that without any enthusiasm in my family, at the end of a usual Sunday School course, I was confirmed. At about the same time, what had gone on must have been weighing strongly with me, for one of the earliest novels I read was *Daniel Deronda*. I fell under its spell and decided at once that my career was to be that of a Rabbi.

At about this time, I do not remember in what connection, in distress, I brought a religious problem to my father. It astonished me and indeed I was offended—I remember that because I remember the tears—when he evinced no manner of interest in my perturbation. Some time later, after he died, one of my college mates reported a conversation with my father in which he had firmly declared himself as wholly uninterested in prob-

lems having to do with religion, that he saw no good in trying
to understand the world in such terms and that for him this was
a closed subject. On looking back, he must have concluded, for
what reason I do not know, perhaps in the light of that episode
to which I have referred, that it was for him the part of wisdom
to hold no discussion on this subject lest anything that he said
would prejudice the evolution of my development. I think that
this may have been so because later, when I decided that I would
not join him in his business, into which he had put much both
of mind and of character, he was deeply distressed and disap-
pointed though he put no obstacle in the way of my doing what
I chose to do instead. It is difficult not to misinterpret what goes
on in the mind of another man, even if he is one's father, but
approximately four months before he died, it gave him the deepest satisfaction, I believe, to learn that it was to be my privilege
and opportunity to work in The Rockefeller Institute.

My grandfather and my father did not set the whole scene
of my early religious environment. My education began in the
Training School of Hunter College, then called Normal College.
After that I was moved to the Primary Department of Public
School 76, at 68th Street and Lexington Avenue for about a
year. In Preparatory School—the Columbia Grammar School—
I cannot remember any episode which had a religious tinge. I
remember nothing that made me aware of my being a Jew or
of anti-Semitism. In a small school we were all friends. If there
were such motives I cannot now, without more effort than it
would interest you to have me put upon it, discover memories
of religious problems at that period. Instead the Reverend Mr.
Hooper and Dr. R. S. Bacon and Mr. Clarence Cook captured
my interest for life in Greek, Latin and English.

When I became an undergraduate in Columbia College I can
identify two main strains. One had to do with anti-Semitism,
though this in a way was minor; the other with what has turned
out to be a dominant interest. Let me dispose of the minor one
first. You could not fail to appreciate the fact that somehow you
were treated differently and for that reason, necessarily, had a
different experience from other boys. The whole of the Greek

letter world was manifestly closed to you. Quite aside from congenial companions among all manner of persons, you had not
the impression that you belonged to a most favorite nation group.
Aside from that I became a kind of professional undergraduate
librarian, both for the little society and its library organized in
connection with the Germanic Department but much more important, Librarian of King's Crown. King's Crown was formed
under the auspices of Professor George Edward Woodberry
about whom I shall have more to say. That racial prejudice was
part of the atmosphere I still believe rightly or wrongly to have
been true and thought that I detected it in my not having been
elected to Phi Beta Kappa, a distinction which I deeply coveted
and to which one of my close and later life-long friends was
elected in his junior year, although he had failed in an examination and my record had been uniformly respectable. Boys can of
course be unduly sensitive, I can of course have exaggerated the
eminence of my scholarship and I may have been completely unaware of the fact that I was an unlicked cub.

But then there was the other strain, always undeniably present,
passing back to Hooper, Bacon and Cook, and still present, even
if not quite dominant. I refer to the strain I shall be calling—the
strain of history. Of this strain I take literature to be a part. For
literature after all, when it is not esoteric, a deformed thing
called Art for Art's sake, does describe the human scene partly
as intellect and partly as feeling. Literature is history. I cannot
imagine how a boy could have been more fortunate than to
come under the influence of George Woodberry. For many of
my friends and for the whole of my life, Woodberry has meant
gentleness, insight, scholarship, democracy and ideals. If he was
a democrat, and thank fortune he was that, he would still have
been everything else that Plato was to his pupils. All that aspect
of life which has meant goodness and beauty Professor Woodberry crystallized. No teacher could give a pupil more than he
gave to us and to me. It was an influence that made of life something decent and something sensitive. Let me quote the last paragraph of his *A New Defence of Poetry* and you will see what I
mean.

And Thou, O Youth, for whom these lines are written, fear not; idealize your friend, for it is better to live and be deceived than not to love at all; idealize your masters, and take Shelley and Sidney to your bosom, so shall they serve you more nobly and you love them more sweetly than if the touch and sight of their mortality had been yours indeed; idealize your country remembering that Brutus in the dagger-stroke and Cato in his death-darkness knew not the greater Rome, the proclaimer of the unity of our race, the codifier of justice, the establisher of our church, and died not knowing,—but do you believe in the purpose of God, so shall you best serve the times to be; and in your own life, fear not to act as your ideal shall command, in the constant presence of that other self who goes with you, as I have said, so shall you blend with him at the end. Fear not either to believe that the soul is as eternal as the order that obtains in it, wherefore you shall forever pursue that divine beauty which has here so touched and inflamed you,—for this is the faith of man, your race, and those who were fairest in its records. And have recourse always to the fountains of this life in literature, which are the wells of truth. How to live is the one matter; the wisest man in his ripe age is yet to seek in it; but Thou, begin now and seek wisdom in the beauty of virtue and live in its light, rejoicing in it; so in this world shall you live in the foregleam of the world to come.[1]

That paragraph gives the quality of Mr. Woodberry—sentient, beautiful, religious but perhaps not quite tough-minded. His was a mood, right to inculcate in the spirits of young men, a treasure to be guarded for life, an occasion for deep personal devotion. I should not willingly have done without what I received from George Woodberry in my march down the years.

James Harvey Robinson painted in the background of my mind with strokes far bolder and of a hue less subtle but far more vigorous. I cannot remember when my admiration for tough-mindedness began. It seems that Mr. E. L. Godkin, Editor of the *Nation* and of the *New York Evening Post*, and Professor Robinson entered my life together in 1898. Mr. Godkin did not

[1] George E. Woodberry, "A New Defence of Poetry," in *Heart of Man*, New York, 1899, pp. 209-10.

tell me to "remember the Maine" but he told me instead "to suspend my judgment." What there was in me to which the second admonition corresponded must have been sensitive because it fastened on to something basic, and so far as I know something which has accompanied me ever since. That mood of suspended judgment is I suppose linked to skepticism, tough-mindedness, and the method of science. Very few men achieve it unequivocally. If you look at a photograph of Mr. Godkin you have no difficulty in finding it in his face. But if you look at the face of Professor Robinson you will be equally certain that it is there. At the same time Professor Robinson's mind, so rigorous, so critical, had room for Matthias Alexander who may have known better about the nature of man than the rest of his contemporaries recognizing, as he did, the reciprocal influences of the mind and the body. For that one was not prepared then as a whole school of physicians is, though on other grounds, now. In that year 1898 I became a life-long pupil and later friend of Robinson. I took his course on the Renaissance and the Reformation then and took it again 15 years later in 1912-13. It speaks eloquently that on the second occasion he seemed to me as impressive as on the first. Many of you must remember him —a not very large man, of great seriousness, with humor of a slightly sardonic kind which came properly from his tight square-set jaw. He delighted, I think, in the evils of the Church which he slew daily with the finest pointed of revealing barbs. From him I think it was that I learned the nature of criticism. It meant in the world of the intellect, no nonsense. He looked at substantives starkly and eschewed adjectives of a mollifying nature. He believed in the mind and its need for rectitude and its power to undertake ultimate decisions. He was the first man of my acquaintance who taught me to read documents. He went in for documents, as you know, powerfully, collected them in books, made you read them, thinking, I imagine, that they represented *Wie es eigentlich gewesen war*. It is a phrase which Charles Beard, an old friend of his and of mine, has to this day, but perhaps in a somewhat different sense, slightly diabolical, often on his tongue. If Mr. Woodberry taught one faith Professor Robinson taught one doubt. A white horse and a black, the two as a team, prepared to draw you through a wide range of worldly vicissitudes.

Aside from ways of looking, these courses with Robinson put much essential, useful furniture into one's mind. I think this mood of doubting is essential for a scientist. Whoever knows Robinson's *Mind in the Making* knows how easily an historian can become a scientist. If Robinson was taken in a little by science, thinking that every time a scientist had an idea it was the gospel truth, he was in a goodly company of philosophers and scientists both. From Robinson one could learn that for an *educated man* nothing need be alien, that everything could be naturally at home. Is it not that, after all, which constitutes an educated man? A man who has, not a bowing acquaintance with learning, but who walks with learning, arm in arm down the sunlit avenue? He does not know everything but to him everything that is known is welcome. Even if Bacon was not a scientist, he was a man of learning.

For some strange reason philosophy was not for me until very much later. Something, perhaps it was the spirit of Robinson or the spirit of Science, wickedly suggested to me that philosophy is the reasoned ignorance of the ages. It took a long time to discover that the reciprocal is the truth. Perhaps it was the dawning loyalty to science which suggested that having truck with philosophy was treason. There were a good many scientists in embryo who took this view at that time. Irresponsibles were made before the 1920s. But I knew no science then. My one course in science was a not very good course in physics, given by Professor Rood. As I look back upon him I know that Professor Rood was a man of great intelligence but I fear he conveyed none of it to me. I listened with closed ears, not receptive to his experimentalism, while the beauty of Woodberry shone in my eye, and my mind was obsessed with the knowingness of Robinson. And so, filled with these things, I passed out of my undergraduate years without enthusiasm for the life that lay ahead.

What seemed the ugliness of business held forth no attraction. I needed something and knew that it was neither law nor theology and so fell, *faute de mieux,* into the only form of biology for which I thought I could secure parental consent. I did, and found myself in medicine. I fancy no one could have approached the Temple of Aesculapius with as little eagerness and as much aversion as I did. I have never liked a sick person, because he was sick. If I have been an acceptable physician, and as time has gone on I have been glad of the whispered confidence that perhaps I was, it was that quality, I hope native in me, but instilled by Professor Woodberry which made of compassion a ruling motive in life. But in those first weeks as a medical student it was chance only, that kept me at my hideous task. At the end of the first week I was ready to resign and did not, only because my medical adviser, our family physician, was away from the city. At the end of that weekend courage returned, I stuck, and have never since contemplated flight.

By what good chance I fell into the hands of a martinet named Ellsworth Eliot I do not know. Eliot drilled boys as an extramural teacher to learn what was in the text-books, not a word more and not a word less, until he led them up to the threshold of their hospital examination so thoroughly disciplined, that none of his boys has ever been known to fail. In that Quiz of his I made life-long friends. It was the largest and best Quiz connected with our school. But the trail of anti-Semitism flowed into that Quiz. Eliot told me he accepted one or two Jews because he had found their presence stimulated emulation. It made the other boys work. I did not know all of this at the beginning. If I had I might have gone elsewhere. I did not know, once the Quiz days were over, that you had no place in a society that Eliot's boys maintained through their lives. The secret of the existence of that society was so well kept I did not know of its existence until many years after I became a physician. That was a policy which did not prevent a kind of friendship between Eliot and myself. When I achieved my place through membership in The Rockefeller Institute he came to me for medical advice and for medical discussion, not infrequently.

I mention this episode as indicative of a phase of life in New York. When I discovered how the land lay it was too late to influence my sentiments or to create bitterness. I had already achieved whatever niche I was to fill. But it was even then a dark segment in the life of our time.

Meanwhile I learned in Eliot's Quiz. Indeed I think I learned there one of the three or four essential things to be learned if one is to acquire scientific satisfaction. Thoroughness, completeness of knowledge about something, the acme of definiteness, a power of meticulous description. One day I discovered about the femur that I knew and could rceite everything about it that was contained in Gray's anatomy. The day I discovered that was my first day of a sense of power. It came to me again later just before the time of taking examinations for internship in a hospital. To pass these, I learned what we called the ring relations of arteries, as Dr. Gray figured them in that same anatomy of his. Another boy, Edward Cook and I, recited these to each other in season and out, in classes, at meals, and on walks until we were utterly letter perfect. That was the most shocking waste of mental energy in which I ever indulged.

In our school at that time this unintellectualism was all of a piece. Had it not been for Dr. T. Mitchell Prudden there was no evidence whatever, anywhere, in the whole school, and among all its teachers, which gave one the slightest suspicion that ideas in medical science were on the march. I should not forget that John G. Curtiss, who was Professor of Physiology, gave a few lectures on the history of the discovery of the circulation of the blood. But not even he suggested the notion that toilsome study ending in discovery was necessary if knowledge was to advance. It seems unbelievable that no one told us advance would occur. But no one did. I was able to confirm my recollection of this incredible situation in a very recent discussion with five of my classmates. What Dr. Prudden told us in two lectures about Paul Ehrlich's side chain theory of the immune process, two lectures in an arid desert of schooling lasting for four years, scarcely made one understand the mechanics of the advancement of learning. But knowing the femur was like knowing one of Professor Robinson's documents. That was a monument of accomplishment— with a past but without a future.

Perhaps it was all my fault—not Professor Woodberry's, not

Professor Robinson's, not Professor Rood's. They stimulated us, or at least me, with a sense of the presentiment of the eve. I can recollect a day when my father asked me what was I going to do with what I knew about the Second Part of Faust. That question of his seems now to have occasioned vast surprise. It had not occurred to me that I was going to do anything with it. That the world had a future was a secret nobody had imparted to me and I was 20 years old. I do not mean to say that like all boys, or almost all boys, I was not a reformer—I was, and spent endless hours talking about how the world could be made better. In the sense in which any boy now knows that research contributes to the unfolding drama of new powers, new insights, new perceptions of meaning, that was all quite closed.

And·then by strange chance, when I became an intern in the Mount Sinai Hospital, I met a strange man whose name was Emanuel Libman. I am certain that Libman did not understand this problem of research either, but in some curious way I learned from him, not directly but by indirection, that everything was not yet known. I can explain this general situation as well as in any other way by recalling that one day William Osler, at that time still Professor of Medicine in the Johns Hopkins University Medical School with whom Libman had made friends, came to examine with Libman a patient whose pulse was slow. It must have been my fault, but in the talk between these two men I did not learn that they were aware of the problems in physiology which the slowness of that man's pulse presented. That he presented a phenomenon which still required much difficult and careful investigation they by no means understood. They thought that somehow in a large jig-saw puzzle one piece was missing. When fortuitously this one was found they gave me the impression that all that was needed had been absolved. But at that moment there were men living who actually understood the several directions in which inquiry must go forward into the unknown, not backward into history. That this was so was not in the least apparent to me and yet in England, James Mackenzie and in Holland, Wenckebach and Engelmann were busily and painstakingly at work on this very strange piece of anatomy and this intricate mechanism in physiology. It was like the situation before the Renaissance. If Aristotle or Galen was silent there was no knowledge; or if they were vocal, that was all the knowledge there was or could be. By good chance I became later a pupil of Aschoff, Trendelenburg and Mackenzie and helped to solve this problem. I learned method from the Germans and from Mackenzie how the tenacity of a Scotch Presbyterian could be driven without rest until he had truth by the hair.

I think it is correct though, and I say this without irreverence, that in spite of Osler's great historical sense he had little feeling for the way in which knowledge could be made to evolve. And as for Libman, I owe him a debt which I shall never be able to discharge. Through him I began to understand what my future was to be. Whatever remained unfolded in Libman's mind, whatever absence of feeling he had for process, he was nevertheless the instrument in my case, as well as in that of many another young man that set us upon a way to gain what he himself could not supply. Later our ways parted. I wish it had not been necessary.

During my student years in Germany and Austria and in England I came to know great men: Aschoff, von Kries, von Neusser, Weissman, Starling, Bayliss, Langley, Sherrington and finally and for me above them all, James Mackenzie. That break through from darkness into what for me I call the light seems to have been a passage through a very long tunnel.

Libman sent me to Professor Aschoff in Freiburg-i-B. It was the first time I had been away from home. School, college, professional school, hospital—all of these I attended in New York. It had been a singularly parochial life. It ended in a quasi-joke. I was born on 65th Street between Lexington and Park Avenues. After year one, my home was on 66th Street—No. 64. When my apprenticeship was over I found myself working for the rest of my life on 65th Street. In a literal sense I have never had the chance to move away.

Going to Freiburg was going away from home for the first time. Whatever else I was full of, it was not geographical self-reliance. I had been told and I wanted to live in rooms like other students. But Freiburg had nothing which duplicated home on 66th Street. The very bath which was offered when I sought for rooms, was used as a storage for unwanted household goods. And so I stayed in an hotel opposite the railway station in order to hear the trains go by, day and night. That took care of a virulent attack of claustrophobia. It was all the more accentuated because in preparation for the year ahead my hospital friend, Ernest Sachs and I did a *Kulturreise* in Italy. Ernest's father, Julius Sachs, after having spent a lifetime as an excellent schoolmaster, became Professor of Secondary Education at the Teachers College. Some of you may remember him—a benign, careful, studious, knowing, portly gentleman compounded of innocence and sophistication. He told us where to go. We walked down from St. Moritz to Venice, aided here and there by bus and train. I cannot stop to describe that unforgettable experience—walking as we did over the Stelvio. That summer took us to Florence, the hill towns and Rome. The next spring we met at Genoa, took ship to Palermo and returned to Naples and Rome. We were young and vigorous. We missed nothing. It was after the first half of this excursion into Italy that I found myself terror-stricken in Freiburg.

At the age of 25 I needed to discover how the intellectual terra-cognita led to the terra-incognita, through that long tunnel I spoke of a minute ago. I had no idea how the passage was to be negotiated. I had not the vaguest conception of how one went about making paths in the uncharted world of an unknown nature. I knew nothing about final causes not being a philosopher; nor anything about efficient causes, never having been a scientist. I knew no science; I knew no methods. I stumbled grievously. I escaped from Freiburg to Paris on every conceivable and sometimes on inconceivable occasions. Professor Aschoff and his first assistant, Hermann Schridde, were kindness itself. Schridde gave me private lessons in pathological anatomy. For some reason I do not understand, Schridde fathered me. When the day's work was finished at 5 o'clock, he took me to walk. I learned the gossip of German medicine from him. I am not at all certain it was not a good education. The honesty, the meaning, the methods, the conception *Fragestellung*—that's what issues finally as a final cause—all these things I learned from him.

The first little *Arbeit* which I did, he set me. Writing about it was my first burst into print. It was a simple thing, but it had for me more than one significance. We assumed there were no vaso-dilator nerves. The question was, how, when it was fitting, did the lumen of an artery dilate. We thought, and thought we found, that elastic fibers did this trick, that they stretched from the outer to the inner wall, not like the ordinary spokes of a wheel but as the spokes would look if the rim were fixed and the hub rotated a little. These fibers kept tugging away to pull the inner wall back toward the outer. By so doing they overcame the force of the circular muscle which made the vessel contract. The notion was originally proposed by a man named Dürck. I do not know, but I think the second birth of that idea was stillborn. It made no difference—you could learn even in this humble way. You learned how to ask a question, how to cut histological sections, how to look and observe, how to spell out the consequences of that observation and by so doing precipitate yourself into a conclusion. That is the method of science. If I had only known it then, I could have saved myself much anguish. I could have known, once for all, that this is all there is to scientific method. The rest is playing with technique.

What it did not teach me was self-confidence. I learned that from Professor Aschoff. He set me a task connected with the pathological anatomy of the cement lines in heart muscle. I collected the hearts at his autopsies and did a reasonably elaborate study of them. It was Aschoff's idea that the cement lines came into existence during life, but in the agonal period. He had already published something on this subject. The proof was to be demonstrated in this study of mine. When I came to the end of my work I could not convince myself that he was correct nor could I convince him that I was. On the last night of my sojourn in Freiburg we both paced the library in his home, arguing with each other. We came to no conclusion. But he took me to the meeting that spring of the Deutsche Pathologische Gesellschaft at Leipzig so that I could say my piece and tell the truth as I saw it. It was an exciting experience—a brash, ignorant, self-opinionated, untutored American physician arguing with the most accomplished pathological anatomist in Germany. I owed this opportunity to Libman and to Aschoff's friendship for him. How could there be a better example of German *Lehrfreiheit* and German *Lernfreiheit* than this experience with Aschoff. When I finished my speech he arose, told the story of how we came to entertain opposite opinions. When this was printed in the Transactions of the Deutsche Pathologische Gesellschaft, what both of us said chanced to fall under the all-seeing eyes of Samuel J. Meltzer. That chance took me half the way to The Rockefeller Institute.

But I anticipate. Before I got there, at least two other things happened. I intended to provide myself with a broad look at European medical science and so spent the summer semester of 1908 in Vienna. I can be brief about Vienna. I was unfortunate. I should have learned more but I learned nothing there except that medical science could become venal. But by good chance I did go to the clinics of Professor von Neusser. From him I learned how accurate a clinical diagnosis could be, if you did no more than listen properly to a patient's story. That piece of information has served me well ever since. I have tried to apply it with uniform conscientiousness. I have tried always when I entered my examining room, to give patients their chance of having their say before anything occurred. It was their day at court. It is a method I think that has worked well.

After a second winter semester in Freiburg my way took me to London. Ernest Sachs had been learning the art of brain surgery from Sir Victor Horsley. This good man and skillful surgeon carried on his researches in a passageway under an auditorium—that part under the higher tiers of benches. This was in University College. Ernest discovered James Mackenzie, wrote to me about him in Vienna, talked with him about my situation, argued him into an interest in me, saw to it that he arranged with Professor Starling for a place where I could work. I did, under the combined supervision of both of them—Mackenzie and Starling.

I landed at Dover on a sunny afternoon in April. To me, after two years on the continent it was as if I were coming home. I was alone but the railway journey through the green fields and pastures up to London, through Kent, made my whole being sing with great joy and satisfaction. It is not that the continent is not wonderfully beautiful; but it is not England, and Woodberry had made England home. I am, I was then, and I cannot help being forever an Anglophile. Had it not been for a certain devotion to American political democracy I should, on Mackenzie's persuasion, never have left England. I found him soon after he came from Burnley in the Midlands to London, at the height of his intellectual powers, ready for a disciple. I saw much of him, worked much with him, appreciated endlessly his forthrightness, his imaginative quality, his utter rectitude, his scorn of meanness, his contempt for all stars except those of the first magnitude. Mackenzie will always be to me the first great man in medical science it was my privilege to know. He quartered me according to plan in the laboratories of Bayliss and Starling and there I spent a happy summer on a badly thought out problem, which came in the end to nothing. Even the report of it was destined never to see the light of day. But this also, as Henry Adams would have said, was "education." Going to the laboratory though, every day, lunching at the A.B.C. lunchroom on Tottenham Court Road with Bayliss and Starling and Arthur Cushny and an Australian boy named Mathison who subsequently was killed at Gallipoli, seeing there other scholars from University College, men like Flinders Petrie—all this was an illuminating and exciting experience. My presence in that laboratory gave me the chance of going to the meetings of the Physiological Society. These men, so kind and hospitable, so careful of the stranger within their gates, conducted me to these meetings. There I met Gotthold Mansfeld and a host of other Englishmen and foreigners with whom I had more or less loose contact in the after years.

Mackenzie like Mendel and many another was a lonely scholar. Mackenzie had had his difficulties in getting his education, but then had settled down to the modest life of a general practitioner in the Midlands. But he was pursued by ideas. One of them was: Why heart failure? That was his *Fragestellung*. He had observed that some women with weak hearts during child-birth developed cardiac irregularities. He thought that gave him a clue to the nature of heart failure. Then he did what scientists must always do—he invented ways of analyzing this phenomenon. That took him into physiology, into devising appropriate apparatus and indeed into the whole machinery and circumstance of investigation. As a result he worked out quite independently the mechanism of cardiac irregularities. This was a simultaneous discovery, the other discoverer having been Wenckebach working in Groningen with Engelmann. From his studies of the arterial and venous pulse Mackenzie discovered all there was to know. This is a slight over-statement but not by much. As an intellectual adventure it was first-rate. What he accomplished is a tribute to his insight and ingenuity. Having this achievement to his credit, however great an advance it was, dominating as it did clinical conception in this subject for at least a generation, he did something more remarkable still. That supplies evidence, as I think, of greatness in character. Further experience made very clear that what Mackenzie was looking for, namely, an explanation for the occurrence of heart failure, was not to be found in this direction. With the integrity which characterized him, he abandoned this pursuit and sought a different one. I am not certain but I do not think that succeeding ventures were more successful than his first. But none of this matters—certainly it did not matter to me. I see as the meaning of his life that courageous search without which there can be no first-rate science. For our time the career of a free-roaming academically unfettered person has value of its own. When such a man exhibits furthermore an ability to search out an important question and adds transcendent persistence in undertaking to find an answer, the invaluable demonstration is made that in conducting a scientific enterprise, the adventure must be pursued in a private mind quite unrelated to the vast technical equipment which has come to be in the public estimation necessary for that thinking which issues in discovery.

There is nothing unusual in this aspect of the pattern of Mackenzie's life. It is the customary way with scientific men. But it so happened that Mackenzie came into my life, that he made of me a friend and disciple and so made it possible for me to learn the lesson which his career exemplified. It was, I think, important. As an isolated demonstration, it is likely to become rare though it will remain true that what is basic, namely, thinking, is not likely to change. To succeed with so little apparatus may from now on be more difficult. It is all a matter of how close to the surface of daily, easily observable, experience a phenomenon crying to be analyzed lies. If it lies so, analysis can be simple—when it does not, its analysis must perforce be complicated and require the use of intricate methods. I know there is a catch here, which I cannot go into now, but I think the general principle is correct. Incidentally the first discovery I made, I made during the period of my association with Mackenzie on a Sunday, in an epileptic hospital. Great excitement was experienced by both of us.

My wandering years as a student were now over. In New York I set up scientific housekeeping with my old friend Ernest Sachs. We practiced, I medicine and he surgery, in his flat and we did science in mine. We employed as technicians two sisters in succession, still friends of mine. I earned $236 the first year and $200 the second. I was responsible beside for the Division of Postmortem Pathology in the laboratory of the Mount Sinai Hospital, began to use a string galvanometer to analyze cardiac irregularities, making a discovery at once—it was very easy—and became Alumni Fellow in Pathology under W. G. MacCallum at the College of Physicians and Surgeons. There I made a third discovery.

Then, by the grace of Providence, having known something, though ever so little, of string galvanometers and because of that report to the Deutsche Pathologische Gesellschaft, a place was found for me in The Hospital of the Rockefeller Institute. I have always supposed it was this way. One night at the Mount Sinai Hospital, soon after my return from abroad, I was giving a paper at a Staff Meeting. After the speaking, an elderly gentleman whom I had seen hovering in the distance approached and began his introduction by quoting—"If the mountain will not come to Mahomet, Mahomet will go to the mountain." I was attentive. He went on. He said, "I came because I wanted to find out what kind of young man it is who ventures to disagree with his German professor." I thanked him for coming. Then he asked me to call upon him at The Rockefeller Institute. That was Dr. Meltzer whom I have mentioned already. He introduced me to Dr. Flexner, Dr. Flexner introduced me to Dr. Cole and after a year I had my place. I was again at home on 65th Street, the street of my birth, and there I have stayed.

It is the literal truth I think that even then I had not learned the one thing necessary for a scientist to know. The word *Fragestellung,* if it were understood, would be enough, but it so rarely is and certainly was not, adequately, by me. After I had worked out the modest discovery which I mentioned a moment ago, I remember very distinctly having said to my friend and associate Canby Robinson that I did not know what to do next. Discoveries seemed to be so very episodic, so unconnected with the matrix or the continuum of nature. What should you ask of her? What is the great question? The great next significant question? I am not certain even now how that necessity for orientation is to be made familiar to oncoming minds. You can learn what it is, perhaps by continuous apprenticeship to a master, or by life in a great institution where such matters are conceivably always the subject of discussion, but precisely what its nature is, precisely how it is to be approached, precisely what question nature is to be asked at a given moment—that, though it may be known in principle, remains to be apprehended successfully only by men of penetrating insight. Mackenzie was only half correct. In looking for the occasion for heart failure, a completely legitimate objective, he thought to find this in the irregularities of the heart beat with which he had become familiar as basic. The tragic thing is that it was only partly his fault that he was not correct. It was the fashion of the day, indeed it clouded the whole of that climate of opinion, to think that appearance was good enough to stand as symbolic of reality. Pursuit of a symptom was regarded as an entering wedge to the locked chamber of process. A step further could have been taken. That became obvious to me later. I spoke to him about this at St. Andrews, whither he retired from London. But he was not quite ready. He stuck still to symptoms—pain this time. But I believe I am correct in thinking that at the bottom of the mischief in heart failure is a defect of some sort in the contractile ability of. muscle fibers. They make up the bulk of the heart and are the motor power of the pump. If this view is correct it still remains decisive to guess correctly on how and with what technique, whether physiological or physical or chemical, or all three together one must set about discovering what actually is wrong in the failing behavior of the muscle or right in carrying on its customary function. A man over 50, unfamiliar with the particular analytical methods presumably necessary, does not make the effort. He tries something else because it seems easier. He has, in fact, little choice, but he misses his chance. That may have been 'Mackenzie's situation. It would certainly be the trouble with anyone who came after him who was technically unequipped. It may be lack of courage, but if you are untrained, you do not begin a life's work in your old age. I also am offering my apologia, though I tried—vicariously. This train of reflection is far-reaching. It is obvious that in the business of discovery the prepared mind is not enough. The prepared mind requires to be prepared not only conceptually but technologically as well or vice versa. Unless the two meet the issue almost necessarily ends in failure.

I wish to illustrate another side of this matter and can do so from another one of my experiences at The Rockefeller Institute. The life and thinking of Jacques Loeb is not easy to appraise. He was always in the forefront of contemporary physiological thought. But that front, like a modern battle, has depth. Even if you are at the front you must ask how far front. Loeb, I think, was not quite there, but he was far enough so that he could weigh relative significance. He began in his own career to attempt to understand the processes of consciousness. His book devoted to this subject was dedicated to Ernst Mach. But his orientation is illustrated in his dedicating his *The Organism as a Whole* to Diderot. What he sought seems obvious enough. He wished to analyze thinking in terms of physiological mechanisms. What he discovered in the course of his life was that analysis took him an almost infinite regress. He came finally to think that to understand physiological behavior you must know molecular behavior.

At about this time The Hospital of the Institute began to function. The plan for its operation was conceived as on the level of natural science, yet no one in his wildest dreams supposed that diseases were to be understood, certainly not initially, in terms of molecular behavior. We, younger men, trained as physicians, were made unhappy. Loeb, the most accomplished, the most intelligent, and, we thought, the wisest man with whom it was our privilege to come in contact, as we did daily in our lunchroom, we thought was laughing at us. My own spirit was in rebellion. At the beginning I knew no way of defense. To build one took years. It was perhaps the most important single one of my experiences.

This drive of Loeb's toward functional simplification was irresistible. It was irresistible precisely because in order to understand anything, it is necessary to understand something else, in this case, what that something else is made of and how it works. What could be more natural than that being caught in the process of analysis from wholeness to utmost simplicity, where to stop becomes the great problem and difficulty. How could you, when you began with *homo sapiens*, come to the end of the enterprise until you knew about the behavior of his molecules? And here were we, poor innocents, concerned with diseases, more especially in man, being told that we could find out nothing unless we went much further. It was a serious challenge. In our hospital I was in the group, middle in age. It was our opportunity to think out the processes of disease. We were filled with a kind of consternation. Being, as I say, in the middle group and feeling especially challenged, I felt put to it to find an answer. It brought me to the realization that Dr. Loeb had gone too far. As a physiologist, with responsibility only to his own intellectual processes, he was free to follow whatever gleam he chose. Why could it not be, thought I, that you could pause in analyzing, at any level of complexity in organization at which you thought you had gone far enough, for your purposes. It is correct that no phenomenon is explicable at the level of organization, at which you wish information. In order to understand, you must pull whatever you are working with apart, a little anyway, to that lower or simpler level figuratively speaking, at least one story below that at which you are investigating. I say—at least. It may be necessary to go down to the kitchen or even to the boiler-room. But you need not go further than is necessary for your purpose. It is clearly obvious that ultimately a human body is a mass of electrons, but it is also clearly obvious that no matter what you found out about electrons, you would not be a step nearer to being able to do anything about pneumonia or cardiac disease.

Having arrived at this stage of reflection I was comforted. At all events my terror of Dr. Loeb vanished. But that particular episode had very great value. It saved me from the view that it was essential to follow along a road of logical, unlimited regress, and permitted me to see all over again, what science really is. Analyzing could stop where it was useful to have it stop, especially in biology. For myself this gave me not only comfort but a new confidence. It is much in the structure of one's intelligence to have met giants and to know that one could live fruitfully in a region less rarified than theirs. Poor Jack need not climb a beanstalk. After all, intellectual respectability returned to us as physicians who could go upon our way with composure; a shaft of ridicule was warded off; life was again comfortable even if it was and needed to be strenuous.

There have been other men of intellectual distinction in our Institute but I think no one other than Dr. Loeb needs to be met on the level of critical philosophy. Theobald Smith and Simon Flexner were, each in his way, men of towering ability. Flexner's was exhibited especially in his effort toward making science in the United States adult. I do not mean to say that his personal researches lacked significance, but for me what he contributed had deeper meaning still. He saw deeply, although he spoke of this so far as I know only on the rarest occasions, into how national adulthood was to be achieved. He is to be compared,

I think, with President Gilman. President Gilman built the Johns Hopkins University with the best men he could find, but he created none. To Simon Flexner it seemed that in science, in the United States, it was necessary to go one long and significant step further. To get on with the advancement of scientific knowledge you had first to educate the men from among whom choice became possible. It is not generally known that he was the author of a scheme for accomplishing this end by establishing the National Research Council Fellowships. That made possible the current intellectual status in science in the United States.

One other man deserves mention and deserves it, I think, with very high praise. That is Rufus Cole. A shy man, if ever there was one, but a man who beyond all others stimulated the study of diseases in this country. He deserves recognition also for another conception. If it were not known otherwise President Gilman made clear that a medical school belongs in, and is part of, a university. As a device, a medical school, like any other school, has value as a method for handing on traditional knowledge. But medical schools following the contemporary pattern are muddled things. They deal so extensively with applied science that the part which disinterested science needs to play often gets insufficient attention. It still is customary, though the rule is becoming less strictly observed, to require of an anatomist or a physiologist or a bacteriologist that he should be a doctor of medicine. These scientists in turn regarded themselves as obliged to think of their subjects as ancillary to the study of diseases.

What gets lost in this conception is that these disciplines have rights of their own, apart from their use in connection with diseases, and that each one has therefore its own excuse for being. Dr. Cole's proposal, adopted somewhat tentatively at the University of Chicago through the advocacy of Franklin McLean, is that each discipline and each department which the roof of the medical school usually covers should be free for its own development, not made to conform to a pattern, but constitute an independent university discipline. It goes without saying that a student who attends a university which conceives of the study of diseases, but of all other subjects as well, as independent

and free for growth and not restricted to providing preparation
for the degree M.D. or Regents requirements, makes possible
for that student a combination of studies designed to serve his
particular purpose. In this dispensation he need not be cut in
accordance with an inflexible pattern. One of these days, when
this conception of Cole's becomes actual, we shall have both
better practice and better medical science—to say nothing of
better professional anatomy, physiology, and whatever other disciplines are tied to the chariot of the medical school conceived
parochially as the place where a knowledge of diseases is taught.

Now I have come to the end of the strands with which I have
made the skein which is I. But before I sum them up again, I
must identify an important one of my mentors. His name is
William Ivins. Ivins is nothing if he is not a scholar. That he
is a lawyer by training, a curator of prints by profession, all this
is minor. Ivins is a fearless intellectual. He spares neither himself
nor you nor the history of ideas. For 25 years he has stood for
me as a barking Cerberus to warn you off from entering the
temples of the heathen. No mythology is sacred to him. No customary way of looking is final. His sharp scalpel is sheathed before no synthetic dogma. The rapier thrust of his mind has on
more than one occasion made me realize that truth and candor
are the property of no particular calling but the tools of understanding, put at the disposal of men who wish to make of this
planet a civilized habitat.

What I have been doing is simple enough. I have been telling
you about the characteristics of the minds of other men because
they are already familiar to you. I have been suggesting that
each one represents an element in the structure of my own as
if it were a building block, and as if I had to do no more with them
than to lay them side by side and one on top of another. You were
to conclude that out of this agglomeration a person has been
formed. Obviously this cannot be exactly correct. It is an easy
way of showing what kinds of building blocks there are, but not
how they are mortised having once been rough hewn. Nor can

it be correct that these alone are the only elements of which one is made. They are only the structure and the shell. What the building has come to contain is not yet obvious. These years of study have provided, not inevitably, but for me necessarily, views on religion and science, on politics, on nationalism. I hope I am correct in thinking they are of a piece. I think they are views that make for peace on earth.

We believe ourselves to be immutable persons owing to the conception that we count on our enduring bodies as being practically immutable for the duration of our lives. We take comfort, furthermore, from the belief that our consciousness is a stream of continuous flow—straight-forward, deviating little, to right or left. We feel secure in the possession of our own undeviating persons—our bodies and our minds. It is as if, having started with a certain endowment and a certain equipment, we are destined to go forward becoming only greater and greater entities. Heredity has taken care to make us what we are. We are strong enough to maintain our integrity in spite of the slings and arrows of outrageous environment.

It takes little reflection though to conclude that this inference is something of an exaggeration. We have taken into the reckoning only those bodily changes which take place with time—our hair grays, our skin wrinkles, our bones become brittle, our arteries harden. We scarcely know even now the degree to which much finer, more inexorable changes, take place in our very marrows—the cells everywhere in our bodies. It is too simple to assume that such changes as occur, make no difference to the quality of our persons. What deceives us is how much stays subject to our ability to recollect. The old conceptions are based on the anatomical continuance of our obvious common sense bodies. We have been assuming, furthermore, that we grow symmetrically when in fact the reverse is the truth. We have scarcely begun to take into account the degree to which, quite aside from the ordinary play of the interrelation of body and mind, other consequences of growing are always with us and inescapable. I am thinking of the influence of those tissues and organs which throw into our blood stream subtle juices. They, together with all the other materials that circulate, make us be and move and think what we are. But these juices also change, in their quantity and perhaps even in their composition. We know that some of them, already identified, subject us to moods and behaviors, often incredible. On the operation of these hormones we have only begun to speculate and to experiment. Personality is not one thing, in spite of that continuous stream of consciousness. The changes in our *milieu interieur* may unaccountably be providing us with a mental apparatus constantly changing as that same stream moves down between the banks of time.

Two other aspects of ourselves come in here; the one is chance and the other is freedom of the will. Perhaps they belong together. But they help to make our persons something less—perhaps something more—fixed than common sense has taught us to believe. This ancient struggle concerning freedom has been challenged by physicists from a new angle. They warn us that chance plays a greater role than we think. The evidence results from their contemplation of behavior in the infinitely small. Out of this thinking has come the doctrine of indeterminacy—if you are going, you can't tell where you are—and if you are somewhere, you can't know that you are going. It is not a bewildering notion and one wonders why the physicists have made so much of it. Indeed it seems almost a commonplace to say that if you insist upon expressing such phenomena in a relatively inflexible language, like mathematics, you cannot describe motion and stability together. The temptation to talk about this contretemps, derived from the infinitely small, as if it applied also to the world in which we have our daily being, comes very close to being incomprehensible. It is all very well to recognize in this the subtle views of Bishop Berkeley, but surely it is unfitting to cast David Hume into limbo when a statistics is still possible of whether we are to be run over in crossing a street on disregarding what even a child can conclude are one's chances of safety. We are of course such stuff as is made up of incalculable and irresponsible electrons, but when it comes to the body as a going classical concern, somehow or other what is true at the simplest organizational electronic level, an aggregate carefully built up in complex structure, that is to say ourselves, escapes from flying in all directions at the same time. It is almost as if we had not known about the gas laws and had not been aware of the multiform behavior of molecules in a container. In spite of all this molecular vagary we have still been capable of dealing with the same laws as if they were dependable forces. The laws have given us our strength —not the incalculability of each individual particle.

There may be a different sense, however, in which these considerations apply. These subtle statistical opportunities which we possess may be making for those alterations in personality which I have just been noticing. The body takes advantage of every instability and makes us the victims or perhaps the heroes of the chances and changes which take place. These unforeseen and unpredictable chances provide the most intricate changes in the behaviors of consciousness. We are in short, not what we are, but what we are unconsciously changing into becoming. The hormones are almost the first little pieces of mechanism that have been identified as bringing about our own insubstantiality and occasional waywardness. Who can say with any degree of exactness why it is that George Shuster can tell us the story of his life as if it were an unfolding flower contained, in the very beginning, all formed in a bulb and still at its maximum bloom and fragrance; and why it is that I was a creature subject intermittently to change, beginning with Daniel Deronda, strongly influenced by him for a while, but ending I will not say without fragrance but certainly not with the one which at one time early, I emitted. The basis of behavior, choice, freedom, is laid down in this fashion. The essence of those processes which makes us what we are, develops very early. It is difficult, probably impossible, to show that we possess freedom, in the sense of choice, without reference to *anlage* and organismal growth.

We are verily such stuff as dreams are made on. These we can begin to analyze even though the constituents lead us a chase that prevents, as yet, our depositing salt on metaphorical tails. One day, surely, we shall catch and, at our bidding, compel them to disclose their secrets.

The need for physical security and, coupled with that, the need for individual security must have been at the bottom of the quest of men for certainty. That need, that quest, must have precipitated them powerfully toward the will to believe. Together, the quest for certainty and the will to believe—something, anything almost—were motives enough, provided there was no evidence that made them wish to believe something else. It seems always to have been possible to persuade men to believe. They succumb to evidence for a belief, even if what they have chosen is not probable. What they seem reluctant to do is what Mr. Godkin demanded when the Maine sank—to suspend judgment. When conceptions of God have become improbable, when this universe is said to be mysterious; when we accept tradition and a conception of God or the universe because we learned it at our mother's knee or from a nursemaid, how can we not be impelled to wonder at our attitude toward reason. Agnosticism seems to me to be no more acceptable than any other half-way station. Agnosticism declares literally no more than "we do not know." But we do know that in any usual, conventional sense, "God" cannot be asserted to exist and that the universe is mysterious only because we perceive that it exists at all. Its origin is not explicable. Eddington in a Swarthmore lecture said as much —and no more. Granting as we must its unknown origin we must leave that origin to one side and merely accept its existence. We could await certainty if we thought someone, some day, would tell us. But that way I think lies weakness. We must on the evidence accept not knowing as final. We must cease to be arbitrary in our wilfulness to believe. It is not arbitrary to live with the insights and knowledge we have. That is rational. After we have understood the limitation of knowledge, living in this dispensation takes no courage. It is full of comfort. We shall no longer need God as a mathematician nor as a biologist nor as a moralist. Mathematical law, biological law, ethics, are the fruits of our own ratiocination just as once was the need for a conventional conception "God." In saying this I force nothing. I

say what everyone knows and at some time or other, in his younger years, has believed. If we but knew it, abandonment of this view issues from loneliness. Terrestrial loneliness, is I think, the most painful of all human experiences. Those who are not trained to it perish or, in their minds or in the flesh, seek companionship of more comforting explanations of existence. But that is surrender—and surrender is not equivalent to knowing.

It is needful in this context to say a word about civilization. Many men use this word in the singular—politicians do and President Roosevelt did. Whichever we do, we are confronted by a dilemma of major proportions. In recent years there have been several reasons for discovering the unitary nature of this world. One of the consequences or one of the by-products, in any case, one of the penalties is the discovery that other people have civilizations as well as have we Mediterraneans. Chien Lung was surprised to learn there were any, except Chinese, and when he discovered his error, he solved the resulting Chinese problem at once by writing to George III that the Chinese had no need and no use for these others. Mr. H. G. Wells will not be the last to bid us put considerate values on other civilizations. We have with regrettable exceptions learned to get along, one religion, almost the equivalent of a civilization, beside another, without bloodshed. And yet, if our religion is "correct," why is it not a duty, men have said, to force it on other men, being as it were our brothers' keepers. Perhaps we do not because we have learned not tolerance, but the inadequacy of our particular possession. We are no longer convinced of the exclusive value of our own possession. Indeed, we do more than suspect that it has not that value. We do not believe a final view any longer, strongly enough to die or to ask anyone else to die for it, containing as all such views do, beliefs partly forgotten and certainly only partly accepted. If that were not so, no one probably would have thought it necessary to bring to our notice the conception—the will to believe.

But we still have our dilemma—the discovery that many civilizations co-exist, on a planet struggling to be One World. We have resolved not to do away with any but to learn to estimate the values of each. No conscious sense of destiny has brought about so much diversity. That is why the way along which we have come, each people in its own manner, forbids the destruction of what we now begin to perceive are contributions to a general pool. No one has a plan of dealing with the insistent nationalistic diversities which confront us. Nor are we prepared to face a future in which such enterprises can multiply. No one seems seriously to have faced this dilemma—asking exuberant pluralism to bow to reasonable multiplicity or more difficult still, to a cold intellectual monism. The historical way may still be best—to worry along in a pseudo-united world until we learn what these multitudinous cultures provide. After what appears endless time these diverse and often antagonistic crystallizations may go into a complex solution. Meanwhile the problem persists. Unfortunately it is not in us to leave to nature and time such heterogeneous elements, unthought through and unarranged. Being ourselves part of nature, we have Brownian motion. But we have more too. And we are, in a way, Prometheans. We have what physical chemists call valences, and valences are not merely passive. Motion will make others and our civilizations confront each other. We may even find ourselves trying conclusions. We shall find that multiplicity of languages has disadvantages, especially when we wish other men to make the effort to understand us. We shall be confronted with the difficulty of learning how many languages we can or must do with, in One World. The Irish, the Chinese, the Jews, are revamping theirs by sheer arbitrary *tours-de-force.*

Can we limit their number or should we accord intercommunicating status to all these revamped languages? Will reconstituted nations disclose in them new penetrating insights or repeat back merely the old things they have been learning from us? They do not themselves know as yet the new things they pray they may have to tell us. We are asked to have patience and perhaps faith. The dynamism of an old culture, expressed in an ancient language, when it is revamped, we are given to understand, will reveal new things. Continuity, once re-established, will have the vitality for creating novelty. We must perforce wait. The wait may be worth the delay if, in delay, we get on with the world's new business. One is entitled to hope that the world will be advantaged more than were the workers who talked themselves into idleness in building the Tower of Babel.

What are we to do with these new nationalistic and linguistic possessions? Examine them, of course. That is plain duty. But we have a choice—we can assert the value of each one separately and so foster and bolster particularization; or try to group them and so to simplify the process of assimilation. But how? We need have no fear. Geography and race and sex and ability will determine the extent of global unity. No doubt we will accept what is practicable.

A pyramid, a synagogue, a temple, a church or a mosque— these are symbols of what were once first-rate solutions, but they remain over in today's world as *ad hoc* evidence of unwillingness or inability to accept later evidence of our best reason. A mother's knee, the nursemaid's tale still triumph. Having once been capitalized as pyramids, synagogues, temples, churches and mosques, many men less scrupulous, possessing a strong impulse for power, fearful of the mob, utilize the need of other men's quest for certainty to protect, as they think, the current political structure as an alternative for chaos. These are the priests in every age. Such motives can scarcely be substitutes for the use of reason— of the best mental power that the best of us are capable of. These are the methods and arts of opportunists and politicians. They have too pragmatic a feel. What is solved wrong, without due regard to fact or nature, is too quickly, too impermanently solved. I have not for myself had time for the "good enough," believing that the good enough cannot endure.

I have, I think, in these remarks anticipated my answer to your question—What of religion? But a word first by way of definition. Religion, as a word, is a vehicle of ideas. Its meaning has a history. It resembles, I think, what can be illustrated by another word, like electron. The word electron is an ancient

Greek word. As its use has evolved, although its meaning was always more or less precise, that original meaning has been metamorphosed and connotes something else now. So has the word religion. Religion can have meant one thing 2500 years ago, but something quite different now. It is worth examining the degree in which the two definitions, then and now, are identical and the degree in which they differ. If they differ, I should not want the modern definition of the ancient form to bear a freight of meaning carried from a dim and remote past. It may turn out that the current meaning for many serious people still connotes something of importance for them, still has a fading comfort. For the hard, rational mind, new visions or interpretations of nature have superseded the ancient meanings. The ancient meanings remain to embarrass the free roaming minds of modern men. Let me now be specific. These ancient devices, religions or philosophies, providing satisfying solutions, were effectual as cogent explanations long before contemporary problems were conceived or formulated. Now, evidence is demanded. I must oversimplify the primitive situations in which early religions made this effort. Surely it cannot be otherwise than that the need is insistent and urgent to explain the world. We ask the ultimate, ontological questions still—in vain. Earlier peoples must have sought straight-forward cosmological answers when they settled into agricultural life. And later, when business was being established, rules of conduct were needed. It cannot have been otherwise than that some men devoted themselves especially to finding answers to these simple but unavoidable curiosities. The rest of the functions attendant on primitive religion came along on the heels of these two questions—cosmological and ethical.

Somebody beginning early but going on to Isaac Newton has always seemed to understand that there is need for the maintenance of order, a need of gods to appeal to, of personal shepherds, of aid and comfort, for uninstructed men in a fearsome world. Special people were needed who understood the rules of propitiation more certainly than the rest. Such men, when found and trained, exacted *quid pro quo* for knowing and for imparting knowledge. Now this is a system which the world everywhere

seems somehow to have worked out for itself with variations depending upon climate and economic geography. It is not surprising
that the system became embroidered and that many men, still as
simple as our remote ancestors, have the same needs now as they
had then. I think it was Ralph Adams Cram who admitted that
homo sapiens was a good thing, but feared there have not yet been
many.

But this is not the picture of religion which William James
and other equally sensitive and sophisticated men think they need
now. These are friendly men, warm hearted, lovers of their
kind, lovers of life, lovers of their society. These loves are so
deeply and abundantly available they flow out involuntarily and
become intuitions—convictions of the existence of God, the will
to believe that he is good, and a profound wish to go on to a
better afterworld. The justification for this belief is no more
than that it should be true. Such men should in very fact, be,
as James wishes them to be, free to believe. In this position,
not fully reasoned out, they have always been challenged by
other men equally convinced of some other faith, who felt with
equal passionateness, what they chose to believe must be true.
I fancy it could not occur until untrained people had fought
each other to a standstill, or until intellectuals had thought
through answers to a great number of questions and decided
that neither reasonable cosmology nor reasonable ethics can be
established in this emotional way, that the timid notion of tolerance, which is both a plea and an attack, came into being. Exploration by rational methods moved the universe away from
comprehension by intuition.

For believers, the ancient definition of religion has been
watered down to noble emotion. Far on the other end of the
spectrum are the illuminati and cognescenti. For them physics,
chemistry, biology and cosmology suffice. Knowledge of physical
behavior, they have concluded, is enough to live by. And yet
this antithesis, religion and natural science, is not a divide with
the soft-hearted on one side and the tough-minded on the other.
A few of the soft-hearted are to be found among the cognescenti,
but some hard-headed ones with the intuitives. Much more needs

to be known about the tough-minded than we know now. Men, intellectually as powerful as Tycho Brahe and Isaac Newton and Professor Jeans and Professor Eddington, to say nothing of a host of men still living, thoroughly familiar with current scientific thinking, remain quasi-religious. Is it because of deep unrecognized and nostalgic attachment to the loves of childhood, mothers, governesses and nurses, who planted in them quite without design, and as if it were pure natural expression, something—a belief from which they have not been able to escape; something to which in the last moments they find themselves necessitated to return; something, because of the warmth of early promises they wish to preserve as insurance against that essential loneliness which brings dread to the hardiest of us as, in our old age, we approach the great unknown?

A great difficulty lies here for men, not able to cut the silver cord which runs like a labyrinthian thread through all the viscissitudes of life, tying the old world to the new or, better perhaps, chaining the new world with many a sympathy of the mind and of the spirit and of the flesh, to the old. These are the bonds that Copernicus, Galilei, Huxley, Leibnitz and now men like Planck and Hermann Weyl have cut without a second thought. The soft-hearted—I mean no disrespect—cling to the *word* religion almost without an effort at definition. For the tough-minded neither the word nor its content so much as emerges in consciousness. If James does not say exactly that believing is fun, he sees in its exercise no great harm. In a dangerous world the chance is worth taking that there is value here. It is a beguiling position. It tries to persuade you that you lose too much if you do not come along. But if, like Clifford, you stick to what you can prove, what seems strange is, when there is so much that can be proved, how strong the temptation is to be content, nevertheless, to be tied to the ancestors, instead of relying upon what is so much more secure in the world of fact.

But James, I think, underestimated the dangers. He did not live long enough to notice the recrudescence of belief in nationalism, all but dead, and in cultures, all but dying, and in religious expressions, which manage to live for no better reason than that

they could be covered with the glowing but insubstantial mantles
of the past. He did not see, and many of us who survive him
do not see, that because of misinterpretations which can be righted
with firmness, fair reason and with patience, we bring new bloodshed upon our world. We do not content ourselves, some of
us, with acknowledging fact born of hard-headedness as the basis
and the illumination of life. These two strains, 1. maintenance
of ancient beliefs against 2. the emergence of a new ethics wrung
from fact, have been finding it difficult to achieve accommodation. But between the traditional past and the rational future
we must choose. The choice is much simpler for those who remain
Believers than for those who insist upon pursuing the new Learning. It comes precisely to this however—those who learn will
be moving forward, though their march is precarious and their
direction changes whenever winds of doctrine blow from new
quarters.

I have done. I have come, you may think, a long way from
Daniel Deronda. I have found gentleness and faith in Woodberry, historical significance in Robinson, scientific imagination
in Mackenzie, scientific dogmatism in Loeb, and critical fearlessness in Ivins—they have been the rods in my fasces. I have insisted that there are no certain guides—neither thought nor feeling—and neither in isolation. I am willing, indeed I am eager,
to bridge the parallel between mind and body and insist that a
bridge is necessary now, so that we deal with a complete man.
But even complete men differ in temperament. I have delayed
until the very end proposing a definition of the word spiritual.
I call it the No Man's Land between reason and unreason—
between reason and emotion. Feeling and emotion—no one
doubts their existence nor the power of their operation. They
function. That is not the question. The question is how do they
do this best—unfettered or unguided by reason, when this is
appropriate? It would be my choice not to trust to feeling until
reason in this region of reflection has failed in its place. There has
been much feeling. Feeling has not saved us. There has been

little reason. Reason is still young. In behavior, in nature, and in the contemplation of destiny I am for the use of reason to seek and to test evidence.[2]

These are large problems with which men of the most towering intellect have dealt. If I have dealt with them I have done so in seriousness, with the utmost humility. I have dealt with them because these are problems with which, in declaring one's beliefs, one cannot avoid dealing. In the face of the literatures of many races, and of profound thinkers in history, science and philosophy—to do this is nevertheless something of an impertinence in a person who has so little expert familiarity, as have I, with

---

[2] Since the possibility of misunderstanding exists, I should make clear that "reason" and "rational" may mean different things. I use the word "rational" to indicate a consistent, complete, systematic description of the world, such as can be found, for example, in the philosophies of the Schoolmen. Such descriptions are rational but not in the sense of being verifiable, as is a proposal in physics or chemistry or physiology. The word "reason" is applicable to the method familiar in experimental science. The world may, one of these days, yield a systematic description, using the methods of science, when enough of nature has been investigated by this means to permit joining the pieces together. Reason as the process of rigorous testing of the mechanisms or pieces of evidence which underlie obvious occurrences, certainly is not yet in position to supply such a description. It is premature, furthermore, to extend what is known of the behavior of an atom to the world of psychology. To make this attempt is to stretch the success of analysis in atomic physics far beyond what a system so, relatively speaking, simple permits.

The word "feeling" also presents great difficulty and a need for clarifica-tion. What feeling means is far from simple or obvious. Opinions differ in the first place on how a feeling comes into being. It may be primary, a datum in consciousness having its roots in experience—be derived, so to speak, historically. This is orientation to the past. In the future, as a basis for action, feeling may determine (sic) a choice dependent on a color, derived from a residue in consciousness, of things already lived. But it can also be a state—a physiological state—which has a background in experience. This (latter) is the more difficult conception. How one comes to be possessed of such a state is unclear. It requires, for comprehension, insight into the nature of many mechanisms and of personality.

There are those, and they are naturally psychologists, who urge the dominant value of feeling—there is of course no doubt of its existence and its influence—as occupying a place in action—perhaps the chief place—without troubling too carefully to decide or to define its nature and its place in the scheme of things. Not being in position yet to do this, creates in the advocates of feeling as dominant, a sense of frustration, with consequences for debate, not always happy.

the important issues at stake. I pray you will accord me one virtue at least, perhaps only one—courage. You may prefer to call it foolhardiness. But I have willingly flinched from nothing I learned from Professor Robinson. Whatever asperities are my own have been tempered, I hope you will conclude, by the sweetness of George Woodberry.